# SUPERBODY

## The Secret of Survival
## in the 21$^{st}$ Century

Betrayal of Trust (1994)
Know Your Drugs (1994, 1997)
Food for Thought (1994)
The Traditional Home Doctor (1994)
I Hope Your Penis Shrivels Up (1994)
People Watching (1995)
Relief from Irritable Bowel Syndrome (1995)
The Parent's Handbook (1995)
Oral Sex: Bad Taste And Hard To Swallow? (1995)
Why Is Pubic Hair Curly? (1995)
Men in Dresses (1996)
Power over Cancer (1996)
Crossdressing (1996)
How To Get The Best Out Of Prescription Drugs (1996)
How To Get The Best Out of Alternative Medicine (1996)
How To Conquer Arthritis (1996)
High Blood Pressure (1996)
How To Stop Your Doctor Killing You (1996)
How To Overcome Toxic Stress (1996)
Fighting For Animals (1996)
Alice and Other Friends (1996)
Dr Vernon Coleman's Fast Action Health Secrets (1997)
Dr Vernon Coleman's Guide to Vitamins and Minerals (1997)
Spiritpower (1997)
Other People's Problems (1998)
How To Publish Your Own Book (1999)
How To Relax and Overcome Stress (1999)
Animal Rights – Human Wrongs (1999)


*novels*
The Village Cricket Tour (1990)
The Bilbury Chronicles (1992)
Bilbury Grange (1993)
Mrs Caldicot's Cabbage War (1993)
The Man Who Inherited a Golf Course (1993)
Bilbury Revels (1994)
Deadline (1994)
Bilbury Country (1996)
Second Innings (1999)

# SUPERBODY

## The Secret of Survival
## in the 21st Century

### Vernon Coleman

European Medical Journal

Published by the European Medical Journal, Publishing House, Trinity Place, Barnstaple, Devon EX32 9HJ, England.

Dedicated to Donna Antoinette

Reprinted 2000

ISBN: 1 898947 53 8

A catalogue record for this book is available from the British Library.

Printed by J. W. Arrowsmith Ltd., Bristol

# Contents List

ANGLO-EUROPEAN COLLEGE OF CHIROPRACTIC

# Part One:
# Why You Need A Superbody

We spend more on health care than ever before but people are now far more likely to fall ill than they were a generation ago.

A major survey showed that today 95% of the population are ill at least once a fortnight. The commonest illnesses are coughs, colds, sore throats, sinus troubles and chest infections. The biggest and healthiest industry in the world is the one which makes and markets pills and potions designed to help us stay well and get better when we fall ill.

Infectious diseases are commoner today than at any time in living memory: diseases as varied as pneumonia and tuberculosis are becoming commoner and are killing more people than they did a decade ago. But they are not the only cause of death and serious illness to be on the rise. And they are not the only cause of death and serious illness to be rising because of damaged immune systems. Our susceptibility to cancer is also increasing as our immune systems become weaker.

*** 

Part Two of *Superbody* explains why and how our bodies are under siege and why the incidence of cancer and infectious disease is rising rapidly (and likely to continue rising).

I first forecast that infectious diseases were becoming resistant to antibiotics a quarter of a century ago. Since then the situation has steadily worsened. I believe that it is now too late for the medical profession to reverse the situation. Infectious diseases are coming back in a big way. There are a number of reasons for this and little that you and I (or, indeed, anyone else) can now do to alter this tragic state of affairs. Our vulnerability is increased because our immune systems are weakened by stress, poor diet and too many drugs.

The incidence of cancer is also rising dramatically – and all the evidence suggests that it is going to continue to rise. We are constantly exposed to carcinogenic hazards (even in the food we eat) and our weakened immune systems make us more vulnerable to cancer than any of our ancestors ever were.

We have polluted our environment in every conceivable way– using it as a global rubbish dump. Most people in the developed world eat too much food but are malnourished. The food they eat is fatty, full of additives and chemicals and often poor in vitamins and minerals. Even the drinking water which comes out of our taps is often heavily polluted with chemicals.

The air we breathe is frequently polluted. The land upon which we walk is polluted. The sea is polluted. And we surround ourselves with equipment – for example, our mobile telephones – which may appear to make our lives easier but which, in reality, may damage our health.

Our bodies, weakened by poor food and too much stress, simply cannot cope with the enormous quantities of pollutants and contaminants.

*** 

The Action Plan in Part Three of *Superbody* explains exactly how you can protect yourself against these, and other threats.

First, you can reduce your chances of developing cancer or acquiring a potentially deadly infection by learning how to avoid, and how to protect yourself against, external threats.

Secondly, you can improve your body's ability to survive external threats by improving the strength, efficiency and effectiveness of your body's natural immune system.

A healthy immune system – the key to a superbody – won't simply protect you against infection but will also prove to be an

ANGLO-EUROPEAN COLLEGE OF CHIROPRACTIC

essential factor in your body's ability to fight off all other diseases – including cancer.

However hard you try it isn't possible to avoid all the external dangers and pollutants which threaten you. Our environment is now irretrievably polluted.

But there is a great deal that you can do to protect yourself, to strengthen your immune system and to improve your body's ability to protect itself against threats such as infective organisms and carcinogens. For example, by taking care over the foods you choose to eat and by strengthening your mind you can dramatically improve your ability to fight off potentially lethal hazards.

# Part Two: Why Infections And Cancer Are Getting Commoner

In this part of *Superbody* I intend to explain why there has, in recent years, been an increase in the incidence of cancer and infectious disease and why the incidence of these diseases is set to explode in the next few years.

Why have we become such weedy, sniffling, never-wells? Why are we so prone to coughs and colds? Why is it that most people seem to get two or three colds every winter – and a never ending sniffle in between? Why are so many children constantly ill? Why are more and more people dying from infectious diseases? Why do antibiotics seem to have stopped working?

## 1. Central Heating and Air Conditioning

First, we can blame the engineers whose inventive genius gave us air conditioning and central heating. To help keep our buildings warm – and prevent the loss of expensively produced heat – they devised ways to send air circulating round and round and round again.

In the harsh old days before central heating and air conditioning bugs were killed by the cold. When someone sneezed his germs died a quick death. But these days our bugs have a wonderful life! Modern buildings are designed to spread colds and flu speedily and effectively. When someone in one room sneezes his or her bugs are kept at a stable temperature for hours and circulated throughout the whole building! Is it any surprise that within 24 hours everyone else in the building is sneezing? If we'd wanted to design a perfect breeding ground for bugs we couldn't have done better than design a modern centrally-heated building.

It's undoubtedly very nice to wake up and find the temperature in your bedroom comfortable and cosy. It's nice to be able to wander around naked in January. It's nice to work in shirtsleeves or a summer blouse in mid-winter. But there's a price to pay for this luxury. When you go out from a hot building into cold winter air your body has to struggle to cope with the dramatic temperature difference.

Our ancestors were hardy and better able to cope with the ravages of winter because through the months of autumn their bodies gradually became accustomed to the change in temperature. Their homes and places of work were often kept little above freezing. To stay warm they had to keep moving.

But today, in the middle of winter, we wake up in mid-summer heat, dash out into the January cold to get to work, slip back into mid-summer when we reach our destination and then confuse our bodies again at lunchtime and in the evening.

And then we're surprised at the fact that our bodies have difficulty in coping with these sudden, massive temperature changes and that we seem more susceptible to colds and flu.

## 2. Our Enthusiasm For Travel

The second big problem is that we all move around far more these days than our ancestors did a few decades ago. Half a century ago the man who travelled more than a thousand miles a year was considered an experienced traveller. The majority of people lived in small, stable communities. These days most of us travel at least ten thousand miles a year. And as we travel we don't just take our bugs with us but we also expose ourselves to new strains of germs and new types of virus. Aeroplanes, motor cars, ships and trains enable bugs to move around the world at a dramatic rate. Today, many of our most lethal bugs come from other parts of the world. You and I may have to worry about customs and immigration forms. But bugs have no such worries. They just stowaway in a handy nose and can be around the world in a day.

My long-standing warning about tuberculosis was given added force when it was reported that two women had caught multi-drug-resistant tuberculosis (the most difficult type to treat – and therefore the most dangerous) while on a flight from Europe to America.

These two women are not the only passengers to have been infected while flying. A total of 179 people are now known to have caught tuberculosis (and other potentially fatal diseases) while travelling on aeroplanes. The figure of 179 is almost certainly merely the tip of a very large iceberg.

How many air travellers develop infections which they do not realise they caught while flying? How often do doctors ask a patient with TB (or some other infectious disease) whether they have been in an aeroplane recently?

The most worrying aspect of the case in which the two women I've mentioned caught TB is the fact that they possibly did not catch the disease through sitting close to the infected passenger (the passenger with TB was sitting more than a dozen rows away) but through breathing in contaminated air circulated within the aeroplane's air supply system.

I don't know what happened in that particular case but there is an underlying problem to which this incident draws attention: the fact that in order to save money some airlines are cutting down on the fresh air used on aircraft. Instead of giving their passengers fresh air to breathe they simply re-circulate the old air – together with all the infective organisms it contains.

The re-circulating of air is now a health hazard of which all air travellers should be aware.

One of the main reasons why people are so likely to fall ill after flying is that the passengers on board are likely to have come from many different parts of the world – and, therefore, to be carrying a wide variety of infection-causing bugs.

We all tend to develop a certain level of immunity to infections which are common in the areas where we live. But we are much more susceptible to infections from other parts of the world. The result is that all of us are probably more likely to develop an infection on an aeroplane than just about anywhere else in the world (with the exception, of course, of hospitals.)

The UK government doesn't seem too concerned about the general risk of contracting an infection while flying. One spokesman has been quoted as saying that they had no 'hard evidence that suggests that the cabin air system is responsible for spreading infectious diseases'.

But in the US the government admits that it is concerned and is carrying out long term research into the transmission of viruses on aeroplanes.

Catching infections isn't the only hazard associated with breathing used air. Second hand air has a higher concentration of carbon dioxide than fresh air and breathing in this second hand air causes tiredness and dizziness.

After an airline meal has been served many airlines routinely turn down the amount of fresh air feeding into a cabin and turn up the fans which re-circulate the stale air. It is this stale air (rather than the food or the wine) which explains why many passengers tend to feel sleepy after an airline meal.

(There is, of course, an additional risk associated with this practice. The pilot and crew are inevitably all breathing the same, carbon dioxide heavy air as the passengers. I am surprised that crews have so little regard for their own safety that they allow airline bosses to get away with this reckless disregard for safety.)

It is, incidentally, worth remembering that it isn't only when the aircraft is in the air that passengers are at risk. These days many aircraft spend just as long sitting on the ground waiting to take off, or waiting to park after landing, as they do in the air. Your chances of acquiring a dangerous infection (as you sit breathing increasingly contaminated air) are therefore increased unnecessarily.

It isn't easy to avoid these problems. Wearing a mask to filter the air you breathe (though theoretically a good idea) would obviously make air travel unbearable.

Sitting towards the front of the plane may help a little since on some planes fresh air enters the first class and business cabins up to twenty times more often than it enters the standard or economy class cabin at the rear of the plane.

But even this isn't a sure-fire way to protect yourself: passengers at the front of the plane do catch infections.

Some people may laugh off the hazard of aircraft acquired infection (AAI) on the grounds that there seem to be risks associated with just about all activities which involve any sort of relationship between a human being and a piece of technology.

Such laughter would, however, be misplaced since the evidence clearly shows that modern technology often is dangerous and does pose many very real threats. The fact that there are many such hazards does not mean that any individual threat should not be taken seriously.

Others may try to find comfort and consolation in the belief that the authorities will soon clamp down and instruct airlines to behave more responsibly towards their customers – protecting them against AAI by installing better and safer air supply systems. Sadly, a quick trawl through recent history shows that there is no foundation for any such feeling. Only the naive, who wish to delude themselves in order to protect themselves from reality, could possibly believe that governments, industry watchdogs or allegedly independent authorities will provide the protection that is required.

Finally, it is also important to remember that many modern trains have no opening windows – with the result that the risks on board are similar to the risks in aeroplanes: if one person sneezes in a carriage the chances are that everyone else will be exposed to (and possibly catch) their disease.

## 3. Our Exposure To More and More Stress & Emotional Trauma

Most of us are, these days, under far more stress than our ancestors. Stress isn't just a major cause of heart disease and cancer. It is also a far more significant factor than most people realise in making us vulnerable to infectious diseases.

Back in 1919, when a Japanese scientist called Ishigami did research on the incidence of tuberculosis in children, he noticed that the incidence of TB went up when the children were under stress or pressure, or, as he put it (since the word 'stress' was not then in common usage): 'emotionally excited'. By measuring the ability of white blood cells to kill bacteria (a basic function of the immune system) Ishigami showed that the children were more susceptible to TB when their immune system was not working effectively.

The conclusion Ishigami made was that the emotional stress caused the decline in immunity which then led to the increase in the incidence of tuberculosis.

This was, as far as I know, the first piece of research to prove the existence of a link between stress and infection. Since then many other scientists have confirmed this crucial observation and have confirmed that the greater the amount of stress someone is under – and the less capable they are of coping with stress – the more their immune system will suffer and the more likely they are to fall ill.

The effect of stress on the immune system is one of the reasons why stress is known to be associated with – either as a direct cause or as a contributory factor – at least nine out of ten illnesses.

Bereavement, separation and divorce, imprisonment, financial problems, anxieties at work, school examinations and even worry about environmental concerns can all damage the immune system – with disastrous consequences.

Since medical students make convenient subjects a good deal of research has been done to assess the impact of examinations on the immune systems of medical students. The evidence shows that students have badly damaged immune systems while taking examinations.

Generally speaking, we live in a world where there is more stress than at any other time in history. Much of the stress to which we are exposed is outside our control. Stress is created by politicians, bureaucrats, administrators and others who have plenty of authority but do not need to take responsibility for their actions. (My book *How To Overcome Toxic Stress* – published by the European Medical Journal – details the phenomenon of social stress which arises from sources we cannot control.)

Frustration and dissatisfaction are now much commoner than at any time in history. We take pride in our allegedly civilised and so called sophisticated society but our complex and ever changing world is constantly creating new pressures and stresses.

Most of us are totally dependent on other people and quite unable to control our own destinies. If someone else's motor car breaks down on our route to work then we will be late. Frustration (a major cause of stress, anxiety and depression) is inevitable.

We have created a world in which we are strangers to ourselves; prisoners of the expectations of others.

Millions feel isolated and lonely. Old, simple truths are constantly being replaced with new, complex, half truths.

The bottom line is that although the human soul is fragile it is constantly subjected to great strain.

It is hardly surprising that a massive amount of damage is being done by all this uncontrollable stress. An extremely high percentage of people living in the developed world are suffering from stress burn out which has been created by the actions of other people.

## 4. The Deteriorating Quality of The Food We Eat

Contaminated with chemicals (many of which are carcinogenic), modern food puts a tremendous strain on an already overworked immune system. I have dealt with this problem at some length in other books such as *Power over Cancer* and *Food for Thought* (both published by the European Medical Journal).

Although it may seem rather obvious to point out that the quality of the food we eat has a tremendous impact upon our health and life expectancy, and upon our vulnerability and susceptibility to disease, the fact is that most people's eating habits suggest that they do not believe that there is any link between food and health.

This may partly be explained by the fact that most people are confused. So much misinformation has been published that it can be difficult to find the truth about food and health. The fact that farmers, food companies and politicians have for years consistently conspired to hide the truth about food has not made it easy for consumers to eat a healthy diet.

## Mad Cow Disease

Britain's Mad Cow Disease scandal was caused when farmers turned herbivores into cannibals. It was a direct result of greed. But politicians consistently defended and protected farmers, and for years deliberately hid the truth about this exceptional – but very real – hazard.

When, in 1990, I first warned that Mad Cow Disease could prove to be a major problem (and cause serious health problems – and death – in human beings) I was vilified by the government for 'scaremongering'. When in 1993 I repeated my warning that people who ate beef, and beef products, were taking a real risk with their health Sir Kenneth Calman, at the time Britain's chief medical officer, assured people that beef could safely be eaten by everyone. 'To say that Dr Coleman's views are alarmist would be an understatement,' Calman announced. (Since this senior government spokesman used the word 'alarmist' I feel justified in pointing out that it was politicians who warned us that we were all going to die of AIDS – deliberately creating the biggest false scare of the century.)

When I exclusively revealed that Mad Cow Disease was being transmitted back to sheep by feeding the carcases of cows suffering from Mad Cow Disease to sheep I was again dismissed as a scaremonger. Subsequently, I was once again proved right.

It seems to me that the whole Mad Cow saga confirms my thesis that far too much decision making in our world is done in the interests of institutions and corporations – and business in general – rather than in the interests of individuals.

Details of how politicians allow farmers to feed their animals are coming to light with greater frequency in the wake of the appalling Mad Cow Disease scandal in the UK.

For example, among the cheap 'foods' fed to cattle and pigs on farms in the US are: human sewage sludge, dead cats and dogs, chicken manure, slaughterhouse waste (blood, bones, intestines), cement kiln dust, old newspapers, waste cardboard, agricultural waste (corn cobs, fruit and vegetable peelings) and old fat from restaurants and grease traps. Those who eat meat are, of course, consuming the residues of all these delectables. What a tribute all this is to the glory of twentieth century civilisation.

If it is true (as I believe it is) that we are what we eat then this news should alarm all meat eaters. What farmers choose to include in animal feed is crucial to human health.

**Animal Feed**

Approximately seven million Americans suffer from food-borne illnesses every year. (The figures for other western nations are proportionately similar.)

One reason for what is now undeniably a major epidemic is the fact that animal manure remains attached to or mixed with meat which is sent to the shops for human consumption.

Another reason for the food-borne epidemic is the fact that many cooks do not prepare meat properly – often by not cooking it thoroughly.

But the use of animal excrement as animal feed must be another major cause of illness.

The millions of farm animals reared to satisfy the western world's apparently insatiable demand for meat between them produce an enormous amount of waste. Farm animals in the United States produce ten times as much waste as the human population and an expert working at the University of Georgia recently pointed out that just seven chickens produce as much manure as one human being. In America, where around seven billion chickens are raised and killed every year, the annual production of excrement now totals in excess of 1.5 billion tons.

Getting rid of this enormous quantity of excrement obviously poses something of a problem to farmers. You simply can't spread it all on the fields as fertiliser. (Getting rid of just some of that excrement by dumping it onto the land is one reason why drinking water supplies are so polluted.)

And so, in an attempt to get rid of all this toxic waste, farmers now frequently mix animal waste into livestock feed. Chicken litter is particularly commonly dealt with in this way (perhaps because its composition makes it easier to deal with - and the quantity of it make its disposal a real problem).

In some areas of America roughly one in every five chicken farmers now use their chicken manure for cattle feed. Such laws as there are only seem to apply to commercial feed manufacturers and so farmers who keep both chicken and cattle seem to be able to feed chicken manure to cows with impunity. I have no doubt that this same practice is followed in other areas of the world where farmers keep chicken and cattle.

I am convinced that the mixing of chicken manure in with animal feed is an important cause of infection. Chicken commonly carry the salmonella bug (among others). And so the cattle who eat the chicken manure also then become infected with the salmonella.

It is hardly surprising that food borne disease is now commonplace. Food from the US is, of course, imported freely into Britain and other parts of Europe.

**Antibiotics**

During 1999 there was a huge row between American farmers and European Union officials. The American government had introduced a ban on some European imports (more out of spite than through any sense of commercial logic) because the EU had banned American beef which contained hormones. American farmers claimed that giving hormones to cattle was perfectly safe. But beef from such cattle. was banned in the EU.

Farmers give six sex hormones to their cattle for exactly the same reason that body-builders and weight-lifters take hormones: they do it because it helps the animals to build more muscle. The benefit to a farmer is simple and financial: there is obviously more saleable beef on a heavily muscled cow.

The row, which has, as I write this book, been going on for well over a decade, is simply about whether or not beef taken from cows which have been given extra hormones is safe to eat. Although there is no evidence to show that hormone-soaked beef is safe American farmers say that it is. And that, of course, is good enough for their government.

However, European farmers are not allowed to give extra hormones to cattle. And so, not surprisingly, they have put pressure on European politicians to ban the American beef, which, because of the help from the hormones, is cheaper to produce.

The American claim that it is safe to give hormones to cattle is based upon the argument that there is, as yet, not very much scientific proof that it is dangerous to do this. (This is an argument which is popular among many big companies. It is popular because it is difficult to counter. If you think about it carefully you will realise that you can defend virtually any activity, or any food, with this argument.)

What we do know, is that the amount of hormone in 500 grams of meat can be more than a pubertal boy produces in a day. And that's a lot. And we also know that sex hormones can and do have a dramatic effect on any human body (and mind).

Moreover, research has been done showing that there is a convincing epidemiological link between one of the six hormones used by American farmers and endometrial and breast cancers. The hormone causes cancer by interfering with a cell's DNA – a process known as genotoxicity. It is generally accepted that there are no safe levels for genotoxic substances.

You might think that would be enough to embarrass the American politicians into telling their farmers to stop using hormones. After all, the incidence of cancer is rising dramatically in the US – and has been doing so for some years.

However, the American farmers (and their government) have taken comfort from the fact that although a joint committee set up by the World Health Organization and the Food and Agriculture Organization has agreed that one of the hormones in use (estradiol-17-beta) has what it calls 'genotoxic properties', and does cause cancer, it has argued that it is safe to allow people to consume modest amounts of this cancer-inducing hormone. Moreover, much to the delight of the Americans, the committee claims to know what the safe level is. You will not be surprised to hear that the American farmers and their government claim that their beef contains less than this safe amount of this known cancer-inducing substance.

In my view anyone who eats American beef is playing a modern version of Russian roulette and is exhibiting an extraordinary amount of trust in a group of people (American politicians, farmers and businessmen) who have consistently shown that they do not give a fig for human health or human life. Just what impact these hormones are likely to have on the consumer's immune system, health or life expectation I do not know. Moreover, I doubt if anyone else knows either.

## Genetic Engineering

Science has, during the last few decades, presented us with a steadily increasing and apparently endless variety of moral dilemmas and practical threats. The subject of genetic engineering is a perfect example of how politicians have betrayed us all and are, through their refusal to take on big industry, threatening our very future.

In two decades or so genetic engineering has evolved so rapidly as a branch of science (if science is the right word for a form of alchemy which seems to pay little or no attention to logic or research) that the future of our species is now threatened. Genetic engineering enables scientists to transfer genes between species in an entirely unnatural way. Human genes can be transferred to pigs, sheep, fish or bacteria. And genes from bacteria, slugs, elephants, fish, tomatoes and anything else can be put into human beings.

Genetic engineering started in the 1970s. The technique involves putting genes from one species into another species. In order to do this the genetic engineers put the genes they want to move into viruses. They then put the virus into the animal or plant which is to be the recipient. Genetic engineering is nothing at all like conventional breeding techniques (such as are used by dog breeders who want dogs with very floppy ears or by people who want to grow black tulips).

Listen to the boastful, extraordinarily arrogant claims of genetic scientists and you might believe that they had all the answers to hunger and disease. They talk grandly about eradicating starvation by creating new high yield, pest resistant versions of existing foods and manipulating genes to banish physical ailments, aggression and depression. They will, they say, be able to eradicate homosexuality, control the overpopulation problem, purify water supplies, remove crime from our streets and deal with deforestation. Genetic engineers have even talked of modified strains of bacteria able to eat up plastics, heavy metals and other toxic wastes.

Vast amounts of money (at least $3 billion) have been poured into identifying the human genome (the genetic blue print for human life). There has even been talk that we will be able to clone ourselves so that we need never die.

Moral and ethical questions have been brushed aside as the unnecessary anxieties of ignorant Luddites who either do not understand what is going on or are temperamentally opposed to progress.

But if it all sounds too good to be true – and all rather reminiscent of the sort of cheap promises with which confidence tricksters make their money – that is because it simply isn't true. Genetic scientists don't have the answers to any of our problems. On the contrary they have created a hugely successful money making myth which keeps them in fat grants and huge salaries. (It is important not to underestimate the importance of money in the world of genetic engineering. The world market for biotechnology products is growing at 30% a year.)

None of this would matter too much if what they were doing was as harmless as it is useless. But harmless it is definitely not. Fiddling around with genes is an exceedingly hazardous business. Simply inserting a gene from one creature into another can cause cancer.

Genetic engineering is not something we can simply ignore

until the thousands who are making the grand claims are exposed as fraudsters, or until their poorly based pseudoscience falls out of fashion. It is time that the insane burblings of the geneticists were exposed for what they are. I have been writing about the horrors of genetic engineering for over twenty years – since I first realised that scientists were making promises it was clear they couldn't keep – but most doctors, critics and journalists have so far been too frightened (or ignorant) to oppose the torrent of undiluted praise for genetic engineering and point a firm finger at just another invisible suit of clothes for the same old naked Emperor.

When genetic engineering first hit the headlines, the public was promised that there would be strict rules about just what could and could not be done. But the rules that were intended to protect us have been bent, pushed aside and ignored. Regulations were, it was claimed, slowing down progress, interfering with the competitiveness of the developing new industry and getting in the way of individual scientists keen to get on with their plan for improving the world. It is wrong, say the scientists, to try to ban new thinking or new research.

Genetic engineers claim that there is no need for caution and that only the narrow minded and the reactionary have reservations about this exciting new branch of scientific endeavour.

But the fact is that the genetic engineering industry has even succeeded in 'persuading' politicians and administrators that there is no need to segregate genetically engineered produce from naturally grown produce.

The risks associated with genetic engineering are numerous and widespread. There is little doubt that genetic engineering is at least partly responsible for the problem of antibiotic-resistant organisms. And there is even less doubt that genetic engineering is responsible for some, and possibly many, of the new infective organisms now threatening human health.

Under normal circumstances viruses are species specific. A virus that attacks a cat will not attack a human being. And a virus that attacks a human being will not attack a cow. But the genetic engineers have changed all that. They have deliberately glued together different bits of viruses in order to cross species barriers.

These genetically engineered viruses can then become virulent again. Genetically engineered viruses are extremely infectious. None of this happens by accident – this is how genetic engineering works.

Naturally, the men and women in white coats who were convinced that they knew best ('Trust us – nothing can go wrong') have been releasing genetic material that they have been fiddling with into the environment for years. A year or two ago we thought that the dumping of waste chemicals was bad news. But the dumping of genetic misshapes and off-cuts will, I believe, create a problem infinitely larger than the dumping of chemical waste or even nuclear waste. Genes, once they start moving and reproducing, can keep spreading, recombining and affecting new species for ever. Once the door has been opened it cannot be shut. And the door has been opened.

'Don't worry!' said the genetic engineers, when this problem was identified. 'Genetic material is easily digested by gut enzymes.'

Sadly, they were wrong about that too.

Genetic material can survive a journey through an intestine and find its way, via the blood stream, into all sorts of body cells. And once inside a new body the genetic material can begin to affect host cells. If you eat a genetically engineered tomato the foreign genes in the tomato could end up in your cells. Cancer is an obvious possible consequence of this. Exactly what are the risks? I'm afraid that your guess is as good as mine. And our guesses are just as good as the guesses made by genetic engineers. They don't have the foggiest idea what will happen. But they know that something terrible could happen.

Readers will, I am sure, have realised that this poses a new and startling question: what about the altered genetic material in new types of food? What happens to genetically altered food when it is eaten? Will the altered genes find their way into our own genetic material? Could genetically engineered food cause cancer? Could genetically engineered food affect the human immune system?

Asking the questions is easy. But no one knows the answers.

Genetically engineered foods have already been shown to

produce allergy problems – and to be toxic. One major hazard is that plants which have been genetically engineered to be resistant to disease may be more likely to produce allergy problems. A soya bean genetically engineered with a gene from a brazil nut was found to cause allergy problems when eaten by people sensitive to brazil nuts. A strain of yeast, genetically altered in order to ferment more quickly, acquired cancer inducing qualities. Contaminants in an amino acid produced by a Japanese company led to 1,500 people falling ill and to the deaths of 37 individuals.

And yet, amazingly, politicians have done nothing to protect the public. The manufacturers of genetically engineered foods do not have to identify foods that have been genetically engineered. No one tests genetically engineered foods to see whether or not they are particularly likely to cause allergy problems. The new food is tested when it is put onto the market. You and I are the unwitting test subjects. Even drug companies have to do some tests before they can launch new products. Food companies seem to be entirely free of controls.

Amazingly, the politicians and administrators whom we pay to protect us allow the manufacturers to get away with the argument that it would be impossible to separate and identify genetically engineered foods! 'Segregation of bulk commodities is not scientifically justified and is economically unrealistic,' said the industries involved in genetic engineering. 'Certainly!' said the politicians and the bureaucrats. 'If you say so.' The US government announced that it would not tolerate the segregation or labelling of genetically engineered crops. The US government has stated: 'We do not find any scientific evidence to support the assertion that bio-engineered foods are inherently less safe. Therefore they should not be singled out for special labelling requirements.' In my view this must rank as one of the most hollow and absurd statements of the century since as far as I am aware no one has done any clinical investigations to find out whether or not bio-engineered foods are safe, a bit unsafe or completely deadly.

European politicians do not have the guts to stand up to American politicians. They are frightened that if they upset the Americans the Americans will introduce trade embargoes. (The

American government, desperate as ever not to annoy big American companies, has already warned food companies that if they label their products as not containing genetically engineered food they will not be looked upon favourably if they attempt to market their products in the US.)

The problems are only just beginning but already they are frightening. Potatoes and oilseed rape were genetically engineered to be resistant to herbicide. The resistance spread to weeds within a single growing season. Thanks to the irresponsible overuse and abuse of pesticides, and the widespread introduction of crops genetically engineered to produce 'natural' insecticides, more than 1,000 agricultural pests have now acquired so much resistance that they are immune to chemical control. Crops which have been genetically engineered to tolerate herbicides have already begun to make weeds immune to the same herbicides.

If the big seed companies and the politicians have their way then within a year or two farmers throughout the world will be growing the same variety of genetically engineered soya, the same type of genetically engineered potato and the same genetically engineered corn. That is not a prediction which is difficult to make. It is exactly what the big seed manufacturers are planning. And when the world's single crop of soya/potatoes/corn is destroyed by an insect or plant disease which is immune to every pesticide known to man (and remember there are already 1,000 insects and plant diseases which satisfy that requirement) countless millions around the world will die of starvation.

## 5. The Contamination of Our Drinking Water

Back in 1982 - in a column I was writing in a medical journal - I raised the question of whether or not public drinking water supplies could be polluted with female hormone residues which might affect the development of male babies.

I tried to get television and radio journalists to take up the problem. And I tried to interest politicians in the topic too. But although many were horrified by the idea all quickly decided that it was far too controversial a subject.

'It'll frighten people far too much!' was the common view.

However, it wasn't just the possibility of female hormones – residues from the contraceptive pill – which might be causing problems which worried me.

At the time when I first wrote about this subject I was so alarmed by what I had discovered that I spent over a year doing research before I wrote the article and my fear was built on several pieces of information.

♦ *Fact one*: More and more people are taking increasingly powerful medicinal drugs such as antibiotics, painkillers, tranquillisers, sleeping tablets, hormones (particularly those in the contraceptive pill) and steroids. Huge numbers of people take drugs every day. Not many people go through a whole year without taking at least one course of tablets. Half of the population will take a prescribed medicine today (and tomorrow and the day after that). And on top of the prescribed drugs there are all the non prescription drugs that are taken – pills bought over the chemists counter and taken day in and day out.

♦ *Fact two*: Many drugs are excreted in the urine when the body has finished with them. For example, up to 75% of a dose of a tranquilliser may be excreted in the urine. With other drugs the figure may be as high as 90%. Some drugs which are degraded can chemically react with the environment and become active again.

♦ *Fact three*: After going through standard purification procedures waste water is often discharged into fresh water rivers.

♦ *Fact four*: Drinking water supplies are often taken from fresh water rivers – the same rivers into which the waste water has been discharged.

♦ *Fact five*: Water purification programmes were designed many years ago – before doctors started prescribing vast quantities of drugs for millions of patients and before the problem of removing drug residues had been thought of.

I felt that even someone with a modest IQ should be able to see where all this was leading.

It seemed clear to me that anyone who turned on a tap and made a cup of tea could be getting a cocktail containing leftover chemicals from other people's tranquillisers, sleeping pills, antibiotics, contraceptive pills, heart drugs, anti-arthritis pills and so on.

Back in 1982 I wrote that: 'with an increasing number of people taking drugs there must be a risk that the drinking water supplies will eventually become contaminated so heavily that people using ordinary drinking water will effectively be taking drugs. Or have we already reached that point: and are people who drink water in certain areas of the country already passively involved in daily drug taking?'

Back in 1982 no one seemed to know the answer to that frightening question.

And today I still don't know the answer.

Does anyone?

Are you an involuntary drug taker? Could you be addicted to any of the drug residues which might be in your drinking water? Could you be taking regular supplies of bits and pieces of other people's antibiotics? Are you taking contraceptive hormone leftovers? Could these drug residues be affecting your fertility? Could drug residues affect the health of any unborn children?

No one in the government seems concerned by these questions.

I think they should be.

It may soon be too late, for evidence is already appearing to suggest that my original fears were accurate.

A report published in 1999 by the Environmental Agency in the UK reports that 57% of the roach in one river had changed sex. Chemicals in treated sewage and factory waste were blamed for upsetting natural fish hormones. The researchers found that the fish were more likely to be affected when they spent time close to a sewage outlet. They also found that fish who lived upstream (away from the sewage outlet) were much less likely to be affected. Apparently, the chemicals in sewage which are most likely to affect fish are female hormones such as oestrogens.

Strangely, some scientists still seem puzzled about the source of the female hormones. (Since the average scientist seems to have the IQ of a dead tree one should not, I suppose, be too surprised by this.)

While they were studying lake water for pesticide contamination Swiss chemists were surprised to find that the lake was polluted with clofibric acid − a drug which is used to lower blood cholesterol levels. The possibility that this could have been caused by industrial spillage was ruled out when it was established that clofibric acid is not manufactured in Switzerland. When the chemists checked other lakes and rivers they found low concentrates of the drug everywhere.

When researchers in Germany started looking for clofibric acid they found the drug in all sorts of water supplies − including tap water.

Intrigued, the researchers looked harder.

And they found lipid-lowering drugs, analgesics (including diclofenac and ibuprofen), beta blocker heart drugs, antibiotics, chemotherapy drugs and hormones. They found all these drugs in water bodies and in drinking water. And they found that the concentrations were highest in heavily populated areas. Once they had ruled out industrial spillage the researchers realised that the drugs had come from human body wastes. Exactly what I had predicted in 1982.

The chances are that no one knows what drugs can be found in your drinking water. Why? Because no one is looking. Most governments do not monitor water supplies to see if they contain drug residues. Nor do they require anyone else to do this.

But there seems little doubt that drinking water is now heavily contaminated with drug residues. And the long term effect of all this is difficult to estimate. Minute amounts of antibiotic in drinking water can affect bacteria in many different ways. They can surely have a dramatic effect on the development of antibiotic-resistant organisms.

There is not yet any evidence showing a clear link between water pollution and problems (such as fertility) affecting human beings. But the absence of any such evidence may possibly be a result of the fact that as far as I know no one has yet done any research into this issue. The research would be extremely simple to do and wouldn't cost very much. Scientists would simply count the number of people with fertility problems (or some other specific disorder) who had drunk re-circulated water and then compare that figure with the incidence of fertility problems among people who had drunk fresh spring or borehole water. But who would want to do such research? Certainly not the water companies.

How are the drugs in your drinking water affecting your health? Is your daily cocktail of tranquillisers, antibiotics, hormones, steroids, chemotherapy drugs, heart drugs, pain killers and so on making you ill? How do all these drugs interact? Are they likely to be at least partly responsible for the way the incidence of cancer is increasing? Are they affecting your immune system?

No one knows.

And no one in authority seems to want to know.

Maybe they are frightened to discover the truth.

Meanwhile, politicians around the world now drink spring water, at taxpayers expense, which is bottled at source before it has too much chance of becoming contaminated.

## 6. The Popularity Of Microwave Ovens

It isn't just the poor quality of the food we buy which makes us ill – damaging our immune systems and making us vulnerable to infections and to cancer.

The way we prepare our food can also have a dramatic effect on our health. Overcooking food can destroy the vitamin content, for example.

And consider the microwave oven.

There are millions of microwave ovens in use around the world. Unlike traditional ovens they work by using short wave electromagnetic radiation to heat up food.

But, although microwave ovens are widely sold, widely used

and sit in millions of kitchens heating (and affecting) the food that people eat, neither governments nor manufacturers seem keen to provide or publish information showing exactly how safe these products are.

In my book *Food for Thought* (first published in 1994 by the European Medical Journal) I asked specific questions about microwave ovens.

The first questions were: 'Are the waves that are used to do the cooking harmful to human beings?' and 'If any of the microwaves escape from the oven will they harm your health?'

The other question, possibly even more alarming, was even simpler: 'Does using a microwave oven affect the food you eat in any harmful way?'

In 1998 *The Journal of Natural Science* published an extremely significant paper dealing with the effects of microwaves on humans. The paper, was written by William Kopp, who worked at the Atlantis Rising Educational Center in Portland, Oregon from 1977 to 1979 and who, while working there, gathered together early documents detailing what was then known about the harmful effects of microwave ovens on human beings.

By writing this paper Kopp annoyed a powerful lobby. According to the *Journal of Natural Science* he subsequently changed his name and disappeared. This may sound dramatic but I have met another researcher who examined the dangers of microwave ovens who has been subjected to threats, and whose attempts to publicise the truth about microwave ovens has been met with lawsuits and other attempts to silence him.

Kopp reported that microwave ovens were originally developed by the Nazis for use by mobile support operations during the planned invasion of the Soviet Union. The aim was to eliminate the logistical problem of finding cooking fuels – as well as to cut down cooking times. The initial German research was conducted by the Germans in 1942-3 at the Humboldt-Universitat zu Berlin.

After the end of World War II, wrote Kopp, the Allies discovered the medical research which related to microwave ovens. Experimental microwave equipment was transferred both to the

US War Department and to the Soviet Union for investigation. In the Soviet Union research work was done at the Institute of Radio Technology at Kinsk and the Institute of Radio Technology at Rajasthan.

It was in the Soviet Union that most of the research was done and published. And it was the Soviet Union, reported Kopp, which found that a human did not even need to ingest microwaved food substances to be in danger, because even exposure to the energy field itself was sufficient to cause serious adverse side effects.

Kopp pointed out that Soviet scientists were so alarmed about the hazards associated with microwave ovens that the Soviet Union produced a state law in 1976 which forbad the use of any microwave apparatus.

Here is a list of some of the adverse effects listed by the Soviet scientists back in the 1970s as having been observed when human beings were exposed to microwaves.

- A destabilisation in the production of hormones and the maintenance of hormone balance in both males and females.

- Brainwave disturbance in the alpha, theta and delta wave signal patterns.

- A breakdown of the human 'life energy field'.

- A degeneration and destabilisation of internal cellular membrane properties.

- A degeneration and breakdown of electrical nerve impulses within the cerebrum.

- A long term cumulative loss of vital energies within humans, animals and plants which were located within a 500 m radius of the operational equipment.

- Long lasting residual effects in the nervous system and lymphatic systems.

- Negative psychological effects (produced as a result of the brain wave pattern changes) which included: loss of memory, loss of ability to concentrate, changes in intellect and emotional responses and sleep disturbances.

More recently obtained evidence seems to confirm that the danger of microwave ovens is not confined to what happens to the food that is cooked inside them.

Despite the protective shields with which they may be fitted microwave ovens give out extra low frequency electromagnetic fields which may be high enough to produce lymphatic cancer in children.

And when white blood cells are exposed to the sort of electromagnetic fields given out by microwave ovens their ability to fight disease may be reduced dramatically.

World wide there are now over 7,000 scientific publications in existence dealing with the health damage caused by short wave transmitters. The damage to cells and cell membranes caused by electromagnetic fields has been well known to scientists for years. (Although, naturally, the electrical and telecommunications industries have steadfastly followed the early example of the tobacco industry and denied that their products could possibly cause cancer or, indeed, any other serious health problem).

The scientists who examined food which had been cooked in microwave ovens came across a number of serious problems. Here is a summary, listed in William Kopp's paper in the *Journal of Natural Science* of some of the serious changes which have been identified:

♦ In a statistically high percentage of persons, microwaved foods caused stomach and intestinal cancerous growths, as well as a gradual breakdown of the function of the digestive and excretive systems.

♦ When meat was heated sufficiently for eating the cancer causing agent d-nitrosodiethanoloamine was created.

♦ Cancer causing agents in milk and cereal grains were produced.

♦ Eating food that had been heated by microwave resulted in a higher percentage of cancer cells within the blood.

♦ Microwave emissions caused serious alterations to frozen fruits when they were thawed in a microwave oven.

♦ Changes took place in raw, cooked or frozen vegetables when they were exposed to microwaves for 'extremely short' periods of time.

♦ Because of chemical changes which had taken place in food that was heated in a microwave oven human lymphatic systems malfunctioned with a result that the human body did not adequately protect itself against some types of cancerous growth.

In addition, scientists have found that microwave heating also causes 'significant decreases in the nutritive value of all foods researched'.

Among other serious problems they found that there was a drop in the availability of B complex vitamins, vitamin C, vitamin E and essential minerals in foods that had been heated in a microwave oven.

The September 1998 edition of *The Journal of Natural Science* contained yet more evidence drawing attention to the possible hazards associated with microwave ovens.

♦ In 1990 researchers in Berlin found that all the microwave ovens it tested emitted microwaves while operating.

♦ As far as microwaves are concerned the most sensitive part of the body is the lens in the eye. Anyone who operates a microwave oven (particularly at eye level) which leaks could go blind.

♦ Studies with broccoli and carrots have revealed that cell structures are destroyed in the microwave oven. (In conventional ovens the cell walls remain intact.)

♦ Cooking in a microwave oven creates free radicals – known to be a possible cancer trigger.

♦ Food cooked in a microwave oven may be cooked unevenly – leaving possible 'cold spots' inside the food. This may result in the possible development of listeria or salmonella infection.

♦ Water samples were heated, both conventionally and in a microwave oven. The water samples were then used to help grain germinate. Grain did not germinate when in contact with water which had been heated in a microwave oven.

◆ At the end of the 1980s it was reported that there was an increased incidence of malformations among children of mothers exposed to microwave ovens.

◆ In 1991 a patient in Oklahoma is alleged to have died of anaphylaxis after receiving a blood transfusion with blood warmed in a microwave oven. It is claimed that the microwave irradiation had altered the blood and thereby caused the patient's death.

◆ Scientists have discovered that microwaving human breast milk at high temperatures produced a marked decrease in activity of all the tested anti-infective factors naturally present in breast milk. The growth of E.coli was 18 times that observed in normal human breast milk.

◆ In 1989 the Swiss biologist Dr Hans Hertel, together with another researcher, conducted a study on the effects of microwaved food which proved that food which had been cooked in a microwave oven caused significant changes in the blood. The authors noted that these changes indicated the beginning of a pathological process (e.g. the beginning of cancer). Afterwards the second researcher, who had worked with Dr Hertel, disassociated himself from the results and his earlier interpretation of the results. In a private letter to Dr Hertel the second researcher admitted that he feared 'consequences' and that the safety of his family was more important to him than anything else.

The October/November 1998 issue of *Nexus* magazine reported that a physicist had presented research showing that the human body generates and emits its own low intensity radiation.

The physicist claimed that the human body's metabolism generates its own electromagnetic field. The weak emissions of light which are produced by the body are an outward sign of an orderly, functioning metabolism. This research opens up another series of questions about the effect external sources of microwave radiation may have on living tissues.

It seems perfectly clear to me that microwave ovens should be banned. And any such ban should only be lifted if the manufacturers are prepared to do research which either shows that these original research findings are inaccurate or shows that there are ways to counteract the problems.

But a ban on microwave ovens seems about as likely as the medical profession standing up and admitting that the orthodox approach to cancer treatment has failed.

The manufacture and sale of microwave ovens is now big business and these convenient items have become fixtures in canteens, restaurants, hotels and homes all over the world.

In *The Journal of Natural Science* Dr Hertel points out that: '...research of the biological effects of electromagnetic fields on life, especially connected with technical microwaves, is successfully being suppressed. Such research projects are, therefore, only possible on a private basis while the relevant authorities do everything they can to keep the findings from the public, denying them, making them look ridiculous or dismissing them as non scientific.'

I believe that Dr Hertel is absolutely right.

Mainstream newspapers, magazines, television and radio have consistently ignored or denied the threat posed by microwave ovens. Politicians have refused to ask for these devices to be properly tested. In my experience, attempts to publicise the possible hazards (and the fact that the industry making and selling microwave ovens has never done adequate testing on the effects on human health) seem to have been met with more concern for the health of the microwave industry than for the health and safety of consumers.

Back in January 1990 I warned, in a newspaper article, that thousands could die every year from the effect of food cooked in microwave ovens. I pointed out that it could be 10, 20 or 30 years before the damage done by microwave ovens could be fully assessed and added that I was appalled that manufacturers had not fully tested microwave ovens.

In the UK the British Broadcasting Corporation (BBC) subsequently broadcast a programme attacking me for this warning and blaming me as the source of a 'scare' about the heating of milk in microwave ovens. My offer to appear on the programme to discuss the issue and defend my point of view was rejected.

(Rather to my surprise, my complaint about the BBC's *Food and Drink* programme was duly upheld by the Broadcasting Complaints Commission which described the BBC programme as 'unfair to Dr Coleman'.)

## 7. Doctors, Drugs And Vaccines

Back in the middle ages people were reluctant to go into hospital. They knew that they were unlikely to get out alive. Those patients who survived the incompetent ministrations of doctors and nurses were likely to die of infections contracted on the ward.

Things didn't get much better until well into this century when the discovery of anaesthetics, antiseptics and antibiotics gradually meant that patients going into hospital had a reasonable chance of benefiting from the experience.

But those good days are now over.

Medicine has again become a major hazard.

And doctors are again one of the most significant causes of death and ill health. They are, I fear, often responsible for helping to make their patients more susceptible to infections and to cancer.

The quality of care provided by doctors has fallen dramatically within the last few decades. Doctors frequently do too many tests, they prescribe drugs which aren't necessary, they prescribe drugs which may not have been adequately tested, they routinely give vaccines which may do more harm than good and they perform too much surgery: all these activities (and others) damage the immune system and make patients more vulnerable to disease. As I have shown in books such as *Betrayal of Trust* (published by the European Medical Journal) doctors are now routinely making people ill and are a major health hazard.

It is vaccines which, I suspect, best illustrate the recklessness and ruthlessness of the medical profession and the pharmaceutical industry and the way in which both have helped damage the human immune system.

Vaccination programmes are a particularly poignant example of the way in which doctors can do harm, partly because just about every individual in the 'developed' world will at some time or another be vaccinated and partly because vaccines are given to perfectly healthy people. Individuals who have absolutely nothing wrong with them visit their doctor and allow themselves to be vaccinated in the belief that they are being injected with something perfectly safe which will protect them from disease in the future. Sadly, there is now a dramatic amount of evidence to show that their faith is misplaced and that vaccines may cause an enormous amount of trouble – and do serious and possibly sometimes irreparable harm to the body's immune system.

Most practising doctors and nurses at the sharp end of medicine undoubtedly believe that vaccines have helped wipe out some of the deadliest infectious diseases. Many members of the medical profession would put vaccination high on any list of great medical discoveries.

The perceived value of vaccination is so great that even though I have, for many years, been a vociferous critic of some specific vaccines I have up until now always been reluctant to damn all vaccination programmes as worthless and dangerous.

The mythical power of vaccination programmes has been sustained by governments and organisations such as the World Health Organization announcing, apparently with complete conviction, that such and such a disease will be eradicated when the relevant vaccination programme has been completed.

The principle behind vaccination is a convincing one.

The theory is that when an individual is given a vaccine – which consists of a weakened or dead version of the disease against which protection is required – his or her body will be tricked into developing antibodies to the disease in exactly the same way that a body develops antibodies when it is exposed to the disease itself.

But in reality things aren't quite so simple. How long do the antibodies last? Do they always work? What about those individuals who don't produce antibodies at all? Vaccination, like so much of medicine, is a far more inexact science than doctors (and drug companies) would like us to think.

Vaccination is widely respected by doctors and others in the health care industry because of the assumption that it is through vaccination that many of the world's most lethal infectious diseases have been eradicated. But this simply isn't true. As I have shown in many of my books infectious diseases were conquered by the provision of cleaner drinking water and better sewage facilities. The introduction of vaccination programmes came along either just at the same time or later when the death rates from the major infectious diseases had already fallen. There really isn't any evidence to show that vaccination programmes have ever been of any real value – either to individuals or to communities.

## Smallpox

One of the medical profession's greatest boasts is that it eradicated smallpox through the use of the smallpox vaccine. I myself believed this claim for many years. But it simply isn't true.

One of the worst smallpox epidemics of all time took place in England between 1870 and 1872 – nearly two decades after compulsory vaccination was introduced. After this evidence that smallpox vaccination didn't work the people of Leicester in the English midlands refused to have the vaccine any more. When the next smallpox epidemic struck in the early 1890s the people of Leicester relied upon good sanitation and a system of quarantine. There was only one death from smallpox in Leicester during that epidemic. In contrast the citizens of other towns (who had been vaccinated) died in vast numbers.

Obligatory vaccination against smallpox was introduced in Germany in around 1816, largely as a result of state by-laws, but these vaccination programmes had no influence on the incidence of the disease. On the contrary, the smallpox epidemic continued to grow and in 1870 the war with France led to the gravest smallpox epidemic in Germany history. At that point the new German Reich introduced a new national law making vaccination against smallpox an even stricter legal requirement. The police were given the power to enforce the new law.

German doctors (and medical students) are taught that it

was the Reich Vaccination Law which led to a dramatic reduction in the incidence of smallpox in Germany. But a close look at the figures shows that the incidence of smallpox had already started to fall before the law came into action. And the legally enforced national smallpox vaccination programme did not eradicate the disease.

Doctors and drug companies may not like it but the truth is that surveillance, quarantine and better living conditions got rid of smallpox – not the smallpox vaccine.

When the international campaign to rid the world of smallpox was at its height the number of cases of smallpox went up each time there was a large scale (and expensive) mass vaccination of populations in susceptible countries. As a result of this the strategy was changed. Mass vaccination programmes were abandoned and replaced with surveillance, isolation and quarantine.

The myth that smallpox was eradicated through a mass vaccination programme is just that – a myth. Smallpox was eradicated through identifying and isolating patients with the disease.

It is worth pointing out that Edward Jenner, widely feted as the inventor of the smallpox vaccine, tried out the first smallpox vaccination on his own 10 month old son. His son remained mentally retarded until his death at the age of 21. Jenner refused to have his second child vaccinated.

## Tuberculosis

Vaccination against tuberculosis is often given as the reason why this disease stopped being quite the threat to life that it had been in the 18th century.

But again, this isn't true.

Robert Koch discovered the pathogen that causes tuberculosis (TB) back in 1883. After that BCG vaccination was introduced and then, subsequently, mass treatment programmes were devised with chemotherapy.

None of these discoveries or introductions had a significant effect on the incidence of tuberculosis.

Contracting TB doesn't provide any immunity against a second infection. And if a natural infection doesn't provide protection then a vaccination certainly won't provide protection. How on earth can it?

It was noticed decades ago that in the lung sanatoriums that specialised in the treatment of TB patients there was no difference in the survival rates of patients who had been 'protected' against TB by vaccination when compared to the survival rates of patients who had received no such 'protection'.

The tuberculosis vaccination (the Bacillus Calmette-Guerin – known as BCG) consists of a weakened, living bovine mycobacteria. The vaccine was used for many years but a trial in India showed that the vaccine offers no protection against the disease. Indeed, when new cases of tuberculosis increased annually in the area where people had been vaccinated against the disease the trial seemed to suggest that there might be a link between the vaccine and outbreaks of the disease.

Many countries have now abandoned the TB vaccine – and have no plans to reintroduce it even though the disease is now once again a major health problem.

## Diptheria

Vaccination against diphtheria was introduced to Germany in 1925. After the introduction of the vaccine the number of cases of diphtheria steadily increased until, shortly after the Second World War, production of the vaccine was halted. There was a decline in the incidence of the disease which coincided with the fact that the vaccination was no longer being used. When the vaccine was subsequently reintroduced the decline in the incidence of the disease slowed down.

As with whooping cough, tetanus and other diseases the incidence, and number of deaths from diphtheria, were in decline long before the vaccine was introduced.

## Poliomyelitis

Paralysis caused by poliomyelitis is now unheard of in Germany. But every year there are some cases of paralysis caused by the oral polio vaccine.

In America the incidence of polio increased dramatically (by around 50%) after the introduction of mass immunisation. In some states the incidence of polio roughly doubled after the polio vaccine was introduced. The number of deaths from polio had fallen dramatically before the first polio vaccine was introduced.

As with other infectious diseases the significance of polio dropped as better sanitation, better housing, cleaner water and more food were all made available in the second half of the nineteenth century. It was social developments rather than medical ones which increased human resistance to infectious diseases.

Proof that the introduction of the polio vaccine wasn't the success it is often made out to be isn't difficult to find. In Tennessee, US, the number of polio victims the year before vaccination became compulsory was 119. The year after vaccination was introduced the figure rose to 386. In North Carolina, the number of cases before vaccination was introduced was 78, while the number after the vaccine became compulsory rose to 313. There are similar figures for other American states.

The fact is that polio (like many other infectious diseases) comes in cycles. When a disease is at a high point in its cycle the authorities (egged on by doctors and drug companies) will use this to frighten citizens into agreeing to be vaccinated. And when a disease is at a low point in its natural cycle it is often vaccination programmes which get the credit. This is exactly what happened with polio.

However, whether or not the polio vaccine actually works is, for many people, a relatively unimportant health issue.

Of far more significance is the fact (revealed in my book *Why Animal Experiments Must Stop* in 1991) that millions of people who were given polio jabs as children in the 1950s and 1960s may now be at a greatly increased risk of developing cancer.

Although an early breakthrough in the development of a polio vaccine was made in 1949 with the aid of a human tissue culture, monkey kidney tissue was used when the first practical vaccine was prepared in the 1950s. The monkey tissue was used simply because that was standard laboratory practice, but no one realised that one of the viruses commonly found in monkey kidney cells can cause cancer in human beings.

(As a side issue this is yet another example of the stupidity of using animal tissue in the treatment of human patients. The popularity of using transplants derived from animals suggests that doctors and scientists have learned nothing from this error. I sometimes despair of those who claim to be in the healing profession.)

Bone, brain, liver and lung cancers have all been linked to the monkey kidney virus SV40 and something like seventeen million people who were given the polio vaccine in the 1950s and 1960s are probably now at risk. Moreover, there now seems to be evidence that the virus may be passed on to the children of those who were given the contaminated vaccine. The SV40 virus from the polio vaccine has already been found in cancers which have developed both in individuals who were given the vaccine as protection against polio and in the children of individuals who were given the vaccine. It seems inconceivable that the virus could have got into the tumours other than through the polio vaccine.

The American government was warned of this danger back in 1956 but the doctor who made the discovery was ignored and her laboratory was closed down. Surprise, surprise. It was five years after this discovery before drug companies started screening out the virus. And even then Britain had millions of doses of the infected polio vaccine in stock. There is no evidence that the government withdrew the vaccine. In Britain official records which would identify those who received the contaminated vaccine were all destroyed by the Department of Health in 1987. Oddly enough this means that no one can take legal action against the government. Gosh. Another surprise.

## Whooping cough

Throughout the 1970s and the 1980s I was a critic of a number of vaccines – most notably the whooping cough vaccine.

The story of the whooping cough vaccine provides us with a remarkable example of dishonesty and deceit in medicine.

There has been controversy about the whooping cough vaccine for many years but in the UK the Department of Health and Social Security has, through the years, consistently managed to convince the majority of medical and nursing staff to support the official line that the vaccine is both safe and effective. The official line has for years paid little attention to the facts. Put bluntly successive governments have consistently lied about the risks and problems associated with the whooping cough vaccine.

I will explain exactly why I think that governments have lied to their employers (the public) a little later. For the time being I would like to concentrate on the facts.

The first point that should be made is that although official spokesmen claim otherwise, the whooping cough vaccine has never had much of an influence on the number of children dying from whooping cough. The dramatic fall in the number of deaths caused by the disease came well before the vaccine was widely available and was, historians agree, the result of improved public health measures and, indirectly, the use of antibiotics.

It was in 1957 that the whooping cough vaccine was first introduced nationally in Britain – although the vaccine was tried out in the late 1940s and the early 1950s. But the incidence of whooping cough, and the number of children dying from the disease, had both fallen very considerably well before 1957. So, for example, while doctors reported 170,000 cases of whooping cough in 1950 they reported only about 80,000 cases in 1955. The introduction of the vaccine really didn't make very much, if any, difference to the fall in the incidence of the disease. Thirty years after the introduction of the vaccine, whooping cough cases were still running at about 1,000 a week in Britain.

Similarly, the figures show that the introduction of the vaccine had no effect on the number of children dying from whooping cough. The mortality rate associated with the disease had been falling appreciably since the early part of the twentieth century and rapidly since the 1930s and 1940s – showing a particularly steep decline after the introduction of the sulphonamide drugs. Whooping cough is undoubtedly an extremely unpleasant disease but it has not been a major killer for many years. Successive governments have frequently forecast fresh whooping cough epidemics but none of the forecast epidemics has produced the devastation predicted.

My second point is that the whooping cough vaccine is neither very efficient nor is it safe. The efficiency of the vaccine is of subsidiary interest – although thousands of children who have been vaccinated do still get the disease – for the greatest controversy surrounds the safety of the vaccine. The British government has always claimed that serious adverse reactions to the whooping cough vaccine are extremely rare and for years the official suggestion was that the risk of a child being brain damaged by the vaccine was no higher than one in 100,000. Leaving aside the fact that I find a risk of one in 100,000 unacceptable, it is interesting to examine this figure more closely, for after a little research work it becomes clear that the figure of one in 100,000 is a guess.

Numerous researchers studied the risks of brain damage following whooping cough vaccination, and between 1960 and 1981 nine reports were published showing that the risk of brain damage varied between one in 6,000 and one in 100,000. The average was a risk of one in 50,000. It is clear from these figures that the government simply chose the figure which showed the whooping cough vaccine to be least risky. Moreover, the one in 100,000 figure was itself an estimate – a guess.

Although the British government consistently claims that whooping cough is a dangerous disease, the figures show that it is not the indiscriminate killer it is made out to be. Whooping cough causes around four deaths a year in Britain. Many more deaths are caused by tuberculosis and meningitis. Furthermore, for many years most of the victims of whooping cough have been babies too young to have had the vaccine.

The truth about the whooping cough vaccine is that it has always been a disaster. The vaccine has been withdrawn in some countries because of the amount of brain damage associated with its use. In Japan, Sweden and West Germany the vaccine has been omitted from regular vaccination schedules. In America two out of three whooping cough vaccine manufacturers stopped making the vaccine because of the cost of lawsuits. On 6th December 1985 the Journal of the American Medical Association published a major report showing that the whooping cough vaccine is, without doubt, linked to the development of serious brain damage.

The final nail in the coffin lid is the fact that the British government has already paid out compensation to the parents of hundreds of children who have been brain damaged by the whooping cough vaccine. Some parents who accepted damages in the early years were given £10,000. Later the sum was raised to £20,000.

It is a startling fact that for many years now the whooping cough vaccine has been killing or severely injuring more children than the disease itself. In the decade after 1979 around 800 children (or their parents) received money from the government for vaccine produced brain damage. In the same period less than 100 children were killed by whooping cough. I think that makes the vaccine more dangerous than the disease. And that, surely is quite unacceptable. So, why has the British government continued to encourage doctors to use the vaccine?

There are two possible explanations. The first explanation is the more generous of the two and concerns the government's responsibility for the health of the community as a whole. The theory here is that by encouraging millions of parents to have their children vaccinated the government can reduce the incidence of the disease in the community. In the long run this (theoretically) reduces the risk of there being any future epidemics of whooping cough. In other words the government risks the lives of individual children for the good of the next generation.

The second, less charitable explanation is that the British government has been looking after its own interests by continuing to claim that the whooping cough vaccine is safe enough to use. If the British government stopped recommending vaccination against whooping cough it would be admitting that the vaccine was dangerous. And it would obviously have to pay out a great deal of money in compensation.

Whatever explanation you consider most accurate the unavoidable fact is that the government has consistently lied about the whooping cough vaccine, has distorted the truth and has deceived both the medical profession (for the majority of doctors and nurses who give these injections accept the recommendations made by the government without question) and millions of parents.

The British government may have saved itself a tidy sum in damages. But the cost to the nation's health has been enormous.

## The growing vaccine industry

As the years have gone by the number of vaccines available has increased steadily. Modern American children receive around thirty vaccinations by the time they go to school.

A decade or two ago the only vaccines available were against a relatively small number of diseases including smallpox, tuberculosis, polio, cholera, diphtheria, tetanus and whooping cough. Today, the number of available vaccines seems to grow almost daily. In the past vaccines were produced against major killer diseases. Today vaccines are produced against diseases such as measles, mumps and chickenpox which have been traditionally regarded as relatively benign inconveniences of childhood.

In the UK the death rate from measles had dropped dramatically decades before the vaccine was introduced. Today the incidence of measles is rising again.

In attempts to persuade parents to have their children vaccinated against measles governments and doctors around the world have thought up an apparently unending – and hysterical – series of scare campaigns. Now that there is a vaccine against it measles has, by a strange coincidence, stopped being an annoying childhood disease and has, instead, become a deadly killer.

Scares often consist of claiming that a major epidemic is just around the corner and that only vaccination can offer protection. I have lost count of the number of whooping cough epidemics which governments have wrongly forecast. Governments are either unbelievably stupid or else they are deliberately lying to help boost drug company profits.

Naturally, countless scientists around the world have spent vast fortunes trying to create a vaccine against AIDS (in view of the fact that AIDS may not exist they may find this trickier than expected).

And scientists have apparently developed a banana vaccine by creating genetically engineered banana plants. There are plans to develop bananas which 'protect' against hepatitis B, measles, yellow fever and poliomyelitis.

Other scientists have developed a genetically engineered potato which it may be possible to use as a vaccine against cholera. The active part of the potato remains active during the process of cooking and so a portion of genetically engineered chips could soon be a vaccine against cholera. (I am not making this up.)

Naturally, the pharmaceutical industry is constantly searching for more and more new vaccines. I have lost count of the number of times I have read of researchers working on a vaccine to prevent cancer. Every year new flu jabs appear on the market. There are, so I am told, vaccines in the pipeline for just about everything ranging from asthma to earache. There is a planned genetically engineered vaccine which will provide protection against forty different diseases. The vaccine, which will contain the raw DNA of all those different diseases, will be given to newborn babies to provide them with protection for life.

I don't know about you but I can no longer keep up with what is going on. I have long since given up trying to work out which vaccines are very dangerous and which are just a bit dangerous – and to whom.

Nor can I keep up with which vaccines might work a bit and which don't seem to do much good at all. Does anyone know what the hell happens inside the body when all these different vaccinations are given together? Do different vaccines work with or against one another? What about the risk of interactions? Exactly how does the immune system cope when it is suddenly bombarded with so much foreign material?

I am an enthusiastic supporter of the principle of preventive medicine. It is usually much easier to avoid an illness than it is to treat one.

Vaccination programmes are usually sold to the public as though they are an integral part of a general preventive medicine programme.

But over the years I have steadily come around to the view that vaccination programmes cannot truly be described as preventive medicine but are, rather, a part of the interventionist approach to medical care.

## Vaccine problems

I have for decades argued that some vaccines may be unnecessary and/or even potentially dangerous in some circumstances, and may sometimes be promoted too enthusiastically by both politicians and doctors.

Vaccinations have been linked to a number of general health problems. It now seems possible, for example, that individuals who receive vaccinations may be more prone to develop diabetes, allergies (such as asthma), eczema and bowel disease (such as Irritable Bowel Syndrome). The explanation – which makes sense to me – is that vaccinations interfere with the immune system and make the recipients more susceptible to disease. It has also been suggested that vaccinations may be the explanation for the mystery problem 'cot death'. And it now seems that in cases where parents (and others) have been accused of murdering their children by shaking them or in some other way abusing them the real culprit may well have been a vaccine. Brain swelling, intracranial bleeding and other symptoms of 'shaken baby syndrome' can all be produced by vaccines. However, this isn't widely known – perhaps because doctors and drug companies would rather that unfortunate parents took the blame for these deaths. Incidentally, vaccination damage can occur weeks, months or years after a vaccination.

Vaccines have to be developed using living systems. They are, therefore, usually cultivated in material taken from animals – in cell cultures, in fertilised hen's eggs or in the blood of infected animals. Tissues which are used include brain tissue from rabbits, kidney tissue from dogs, rabbits and monkeys, protein from hen's or duck's eggs, blood from horses or pigs. This system can, of course, be dangerous since cell cultures may be contaminated (as was the case with the polio vaccine made with monkey tissue). Some vaccines have been prepared using bovine serum and it now appears that during the early 1990s an unknown number of British children received vaccinations which may have been prepared using material from British cattle which could have been infected with BSE.

Naturally, no one knows the size of the risk that was taken

at the time (though it seems that the British government was warned of the hazard).

And no one is likely to know the size of any problem resulting from this for at least a decade. This is yet another piece of powerful evidence supporting those who are opposed to mass vaccination programmes.

(It is perhaps relevant to point out that vaccines also often contain additives. Antibiotics may be added to dampen down the immune system response. And stabilisers of various kinds may also be included.)

Evidence that vaccines may do more harm than good is supported by experiences with animals. Between 1968 and 1988 there were considerably more outbreaks of foot and mouth disease in countries where vaccination against foot and mouth disease was compulsory than in countries where there were no such regulations. Epidemics always started in countries where vaccination was compulsory. This experience clearly shows that the alleged advantage to the community of vaccinating individuals simply does not exist.

Similar observations were made about the hyena dog, which was in 1989 threatened with extinction. Scientists vaccinated individual animals to protect them against rabies but more than a dozen packs then died within a year – of rabies. This happened even in areas where rabies had never been seen before. When researchers tried using a non infectious form of the pathogen (to prevent the deaths of the remaining animals) all members of seven packs of dogs disappeared. And yet the rabies vaccine is now compulsory in many parts of the world. Is it not possible that it is the vaccine which is keeping this disease alive?

Those who eat meat should be aware that cattle (and other animals reared for slaughter) are regularly vaccinated. The meat that is taken from those animals may, therefore, contain vaccine residues in addition to hormones, antibiotics and other drugs.

Tragically, many doctors seem to know very little about the vaccines they advocate. In my view, if a doctor wants to vaccinate you or a member of your family you should insist that he confirm in writing that the vaccine is both entirely safe and absolutely essential. You may notice his enthusiasm for the vaccine suddenly diminish.

Finally, despite all this evidence vaccines for children and adults are compulsory in some countries. In other countries (such as the UK) doctors are given a financial bonus as a reward when they 'sell' vaccination to a large proportion of their patients.

As more and more people become wary about vaccines so it is likely that more and more countries will make vaccination compulsory.

## 8. The Destruction Of Antibiotic Power

A few decades ago the development of antibiotics led many people to believe that the threat offered by infectious diseases had, to a large extent, been conquered.

But a combination of greed and stupidity has changed all that. The effectiveness of antibiotics has been dramatically weakened by three main groups: the companies making them, the medical profession and the farming industry. Each of these groups has acted irresponsibly and dangerously. Since they cannot possibly have been unaware of the impact their actions would have it is impossible to avoid the conclusion that the effectiveness of antibiotics has been deliberately destroyed for short term profit. The drug companies, the medical establishment and the farming industry will together be responsible for millions of deaths. The politicians who have stood to one side and allowed all this to happen must share the responsibility.

The destruction of antibiotics as a weapon in the fight against infection is not a reason why we are now more vulnerable to infection. But it is an important reason why the number of people dying from infections is rising – and will rise dramatically during the next decade or so.

During the last two decades simple, widespread infections have been striking back and once again re-establishing themselves as serious threats to our health – as serious as cancer and heart disease.

In 1952 virtually all infections caused by staphylococcus could be cured by penicillin. But by 1982 a worrying 90% of patients infected with the staphylococcus bug needed treatment with other antibiotics. Penicillin – the best known, cheapest and most widely available antibiotic in the world – no longer worked against staphylococcus.

Doctors didn't worry about this because they had other antibiotics to prescribe. With remarkable arrogance the medical profession assumed that it could always stay one step ahead of the bugs.

What many doctors failed to realise was that yeasts, fungi and bacteria have been producing antibiotics more or less since time began. They use the antibiotics they make to protect themselves. Other yeasts, fungi and bacteria mutate naturally in order to protect themselves against those antibiotics. Through a mixture of ignorance and arrogance doctors speeded up the rate at which bugs acquired resistance by spreading antibiotics around with reckless abandon.

The staphylococcus bug is widespread and constantly being passed from one person to another. It is possible to pick up staphylococcus simply through a handshake. It also affects some mammalian pets and so can be picked up that way too.

Most of the time the body's immune system deals with the bug fairly quickly and effectively. The staphylococcus only becomes a real problem when it is picked up by a human being with a wound of some kind – or an immune system that is out of condition or already stretched so much that it cannot cope. Under those circumstances the staphylococcus can kill.

In order to try to stop staphylococcus bugs causing so many deaths in hospitals doctors started routinely giving antibiotics to all the patients whom they thought might be at risk – and this category naturally included all those patients who were destined for surgery.

The prescribing doctors either didn't realise or didn't care that by dishing out antibiotics so freely they were giving the bugs a greatly increased chance of acquiring immunity.

Staphylococcus has not, of course, been the only bug to

become resistant. In 1990 Jim Henson, the inventor of TV puppet stars The Muppets, died of a new, resistant streptococcal infection. Doctors suddenly started to report the existence of antibiotic-resistant strains of streptococcus pneumoniae – which were new enough and virulent enough to kill individuals with weakened immune systems.

Leprosy, easily treated until the late 1970s, became a major problem again when a new, resistant type of the bacterium mycobacterium leprae appeared in Ethiopia. Gonorrhoea acquired worldwide resistance to penicillin and other drugs. By 1990 eight out of ten illnesses caused by shigella were resistant to antibiotics. Malaria, apparently almost under control in the 1950s, has become a major killer because of the drug-resistant plasmodium falciparum parasites. Tuberculosis, still apparently regarded by many doctors as a disease of the 19th century, has come back with a vengeance with the development of a drug-resistant strain. UNICEF is now warning that antibiotic-resistant strains of tuberculosis need to be taken seriously. Tuberculosis kills over three million people every year. I have been warning about the resurgence of tuberculosis for a decade.

Throughout the early 1990s doctors in the developed world tried to combat new outbreaks of infectious disease by prescribing antibiotics in ever increasing quantities. They also tried to protect patients against infection by prescribing antibiotics for healthy patients. Naturally enough the drug industry, which was making huge profits out of the sale of antibiotics, did not object to this. Politicians, constantly afraid of offending the drug companies, did everything they could to stifle protests by people like me who wrote about this problem and warned about the future consequences.

In the developing countries, where doctors were not always available, patients simply bought their own antibiotics. (Ironically – and in my view with considerable cheek – some observers in the developed world are now blaming the overuse of antibiotics in the developing world for the fact that new antibiotic-resistant bugs are now a serious worldwide threat.)

Today the future is truly bleak. Infectious diseases which we thought we had conquered are coming back with a vengeance

More and more people are dying of simple, uncomplicated infections. The bugs are getting stronger. And our ability to zap them is diminishing almost daily.

I have, for many years, written about the way that doctors do harm by over-prescribing. The best example of the modern tendency to over-prescribe probably lies in the way that antibiotics are used. One in six prescriptions is for an antibiotic and there are at least a hundred different antibiotics available for doctors to choose from.

When antibiotics – drugs such as penicillin – were first introduced in the 1930s they gave doctors a chance to kill the bacteria causing infections. My educated guestimate is that for several decades between half and three quarters of all the prescriptions written for antibiotics have been unnecessary or inappropriate. That is still the situation today.

To a certain extent doctors over-prescribe because they like to do something when faced with a patient – and prescribing a drug is virtually the only thing most of them can do. Prescribing a drug is also a defence against any possible future charge of negligence (on the basis that if the patient dies it is better to have done something than to have done nothing).

But the main reason for the over-prescribing of antibiotics is, without doubt, the fact that doctors are under the influence of the drug companies. The makers of the antibiotics want their drugs prescribed in vast quantities. It makes no difference to them whether or not the prescriptions are necessary. There is now no doubt that many of our most useful drugs have been devalued by overuse and are no longer effective.

Doctors regularly hand out these potentially life-saving pills for minor coughs and infections that would have got better anyway within days. Colds and flu are caused by viruses – which are not susceptible to antibiotics.

The excessive quantities of antibiotics we have swallowed by the ton have weakened our general resistance to infection and paradoxically, strengthened the power of the bugs.

The existence of many antibiotic-resistant organisms is the main reason why infections are such a major problem in hospitals.

Alarmingly, at least 1 in 20 of all hospital patients will pick up an infection in hospital – mostly urinary tract, chest or wound infections. Bizarrely, the spread of these antibiotic-resistant organisms is mostly caused by doctors and nurses failing to wash their hands often enough. Since Ignaz Philipp Semmelweiss first demonstrated (in the mid-19th century) that deaths in the delivery room were caused by dirty hands every child has been taught the importance of basic personal hygiene. Sadly, the message does not seem to have got through to the medical and nursing professions. Several recent studies have shown that neither doctors nor nurses wash their hands anywhere near as often as they should. At least one-third of all hospital infections are caused by dirty hands and the cost in simple financial terms is colossal (though not, of course, as horrendous or as unforgivable as the cost in human terms). It is hardly surprising that people who stay at home to be treated – or who go home quickly after day-case or short-stay surgery – usually get better much quicker than people who need long-stay treatment.

By the mid 1980s it was already becoming clear that bad prescribing was causing serious problems. Strains of staphylococcus were appearing which were resistant to many antibiotics.

At first the new superbugs only caused problems within hospitals – where they caused many deaths among patients whose immune systems had been compromised by other diseases or by physical or mental stresses. It was in hospitals that many superbugs first started to appear but by the early 1990s the staphylococcal superbugs were appearing inside and outside hospitals all around the world.

The problem was so great that the extra costs incurred when doctors had to prescribe increasingly expensive antibiotics was beginning to add an enormous burden to all those responsible for providing health care facilities. In America the extra cost of dealing with antibiotic-resistant organisms was, by the end of the 1980s, estimated at being in excess of $30 billion a year.

Salmonella became a more or less untreatable disease in 1993 and now poses a serious health threat. According to the US Department of Agriculture 661,000 people are made ill every year by salmonella-infected eggs. Of those around 400 people die. The Department of Agriculture's original count was considerably higher. The figure of 661,000 was obtained after a recount. I don't have any figures I trust for any other country. In the UK I certainly wouldn't trust any figures produced by the Ministry of Agriculture and Fisheries.

The big problem with salmonella bacteria is that some strains are already resistant to ampicillin, streptomycin, tetracycline, sulphonamides and chloramphenicol. It won't be long before some salmonella bacteria are resistant to all known antibiotics. When that happens the death rate from salmonella will rocket.

Most salmonella antibiotic resistance develops on farms where more than half of all antibiotics produced are used (I will explain why in a moment or two). Naturally, the salmonella bacteria in chickens affect the flesh of the birds as well as their eggs. And the bacteria can easily spread from chicken flesh to other products.

My informed and considered view is that if you are an egg eating heterosexual and you don't mainline illegal drugs with dirty needles then you are more likely to contract and/or die of salmonella poisoning than you are to contract and/or die of the group of diseases known as AIDS.

Moreover, there seems little doubt that unless the mass use of antibiotics on farms is stopped then salmonella poisoning will pose a considerably greater threat to future generations of the human race than AIDS. Nevertheless, I have no doubt that governments will continue to spend billions on researching still fashionable AIDS but will not risk offending the rich farming lobby by suggesting that antibiotic use be reduced.

Partly thanks to doctors and drug companies the future is truly bleak. Infectious diseases which we thought we had conquered are coming back with a vengeance. More and more people are dying of simple, uncomplicated infections. The bugs are getting stronger. And our ability to kill them is diminishing almost daily.

Scientists messing around with genes are making things considerably worse and ensuring that the future is even more bleak than the present.

However, it is the overuse of antibiotics by farmers which is one of the main reasons why infectious diseases are making a dramatic comeback. Farmers are going to be directly responsible for millions of deaths.

Astonishingly, considerably more than half of all the antibiotics sold are given by farmers to healthy animals. Giving antibiotics helps improve the size and therefore the value of animals. I first wrote about this grossly irresponsible but profitable habit back in the 1970s but politicians have steadfastly refused to take on the farming community and stop farmers using antibiotics.

Why do farmers give their animals so many antibiotics?

Well, to start with, farmers give some antibiotics to animals to help prevent (and treat) disease. Animals on modern farms are exceptionally susceptible to disease because they are kept in overcrowded conditions and they are constantly highly stressed. Antibiotics help to keep sick animals alive long enough to be slaughtered and fed into the food chain. Antibiotics are also given because they help to stop diseases spreading quickly among animals who are kept in cramped and entirely unnatural conditions. When animals live in hideously confined quarters it is nigh on impossible to stop infections spreading without using antibiotics.

Many farmers also routinely put antibiotics into the feed they give their animals to prevent infections developing and the antibiotics that are dished out in this grossly irresponsible way are often the same antibiotics that are becoming dramatically less effective in the treatment of human diseases.

But farmers don't just give antibiotics to animals in order to deal with disease. It was reported in 1998 that some 10,000 pig, poultry and beef farms in Britain alone were mixing antibiotics into their animal feed in order to promote growth.

Back in the 1940s it was noticed that animals who were regularly given antibiotics put on weight more rapidly than animals who weren't. I don't think anyone knows why this happens but antibiotics increase the muscle bulk of animals – and therefore increase their value and the farmer's eventual profit.

Despite the fact that antibiotic resistance was, even then, acknowledged to be a problem, farmers started to give their animals antibiotics in order to increase their profits. To their eternal shame vets and politicians succumbed to pressure from the farmers and allowed this to happen. (In an attempt to disguise their guilt – and to hide what they are doing – farmers describe the antibiotics they give to animals as 'digestive enhancers'.) Amazingly, farmers do not need a prescription from a vet in order to give antibiotics to their animals on a regular, daily basis. You need to visit a doctor to get an antibiotic if you have an infection which needs treatment. But farmers can buy their antibiotics in bulk – and throw them into the animal feed by the fistful.

Of course, there have over the years been a few pretty half hearted attempts to stop this grossly irresponsible practice. Various committees and organisations (including the World Health Organization) have recommended phasing out the routine use of antibiotics as growth enhancers.

(I am afraid I cannot explain why 'phasing out' has been recommended instead of simply halting this outrageous practice – though undoubtedly the power of the farming industry has much to do with this.)

In December 1998 the European Union finally proposed a ban on the use of some antibiotics by farmers. The British government said it would probably support such a ban but it was clear that any such move would probably prove pointless when drug companies said they would challenge any such ban in the courts. A legal battle on such a complex issue would, with all the appropriate appeals, probably last for at least a decade. In the end the EU announced with a great fanfare that it had banned farmers from using just four antibiotics. But they did not introduce a general ban on the use of the tetracyclines and penicillins – the drugs which are most commonly used both on animals and for human patients. In my view this was akin to making murder illegal between 10.45 pm and 10.50 pm on alternate Wednesdays.

The process by which antibiotic resistance develops is simple to explain. When animals are given antibiotics the bacteria in their intestines build up an immunity to those antibiotics. Those antibiotic-resistant organisms then pass on to farmers and others who have contact with the animals. They pass into the environment (even though most animals are denied access to fields their faeces and urine still reach the environment when they are dumped onto fields or discharged into rivers). And, of course, the antibiotic-resistant organisms pass into the food chain directly when animals are killed, chopped up and eaten by humans. When milk in the US was tested researchers identified 52 different antibiotic residues.

As if all this wasn't bad enough there is also evidence that the antibiotic-resistant organisms can pass their resistance on to other, more dangerous bacteria. There are already some dangerous infections which are virtually untreatable because the bugs involved are resistant to all the available antibiotics.

### Genetic Engineering and Antiobiotics

In addition to the two obvious causes of the increase in the growth of antibiotic-resistant organisms (the use of antibiotics by farmers and the overprescribing of antibiotics by doctors) there is another reason for this problem: genetic engineering.

It has been found that the emergence of antibiotic-resistant bacteria is associated with something known as 'horizontal gene transfer' – in which genes move from species to species. You will, I suspect, not be surprised to hear that 'horizontal gene transfer' is exactly what genetic engineers do. Genetic engineers have spent years, and much money, finding ways to break down the natural barriers which prevent the transfer of genes from one species to another. Genetic engineering has enabled bacteria to share their acquired ability to resist antibiotics and to grow stronger and stronger.

Even more frightening is the fact that once horizontal gene transfer starts it is speeded up by the use of antibiotics – which encourage the exchange of genes between different species. So, the more we use antibiotics to try and deal with these new and resistant organisms the more resistant organisms there will be. Things aren't helped by the fact that genetic engineers use antibiotic-resistant genes to tag and mark the bits and pieces of genetic material they are moving about.

For a while scientists believed that horizontal gene transfer was something that only happened between bacteria. But this isn't true. It is possible for genes to move from virtually any species to any other species. Genetic engineers have made this process faster and more efficient.

## 9. Cancer Is Often Caused By The Chemical Poisons And Toxins Which Pollute Our World (But The Cancer Industry Fiddles While The World Is Dying)

The mortality figures show that more people than ever are dying from cancer. One in three people already have, or will develop, cancer. The figure will be one in two before long. And figures from around the world show that the picture is much the same everywhere.

Wherever you live, and whatever you do for a living, you are almost certainly exposed to an almost endless variety of carcinogens (cancer causing substances) every day of your life.

There are carcinogens in tobacco and in the food we eat. Many of the chemicals which farmers spray around the countryside (and, more potently, onto farm land) are known to be carcinogenic. Many of the substances fed to farm animals are known to cause cancer too.

It is nigh on impossible to avoid contact with these deadly substances.

Chemicals from diesel fumes are believed to cause 10,000 deaths a year in the UK alone. Japanese researchers who have discovered a compound called 3 nitro benzathrone in the exhaust emissions of diesel engines claim that it is the most carcinogenic substance ever analysed. As a result fumes from lorries are probably responsible for the high incidence of lung cancer among city dwellers.

(The production of 3 nitro benzathrone increases dramatically when engines are pulling heavy loads. One obvious answer is to regulate the size of loads that diesel trucks can pull. Putting heavier taxes on lorries would be an even better idea – that would force haulage companies to use the railways more. But since politicians are reluctant to take action the only practical answer is for you and I to do our best to avoid areas where diesel trucks congregate. The most dangerous spots are probably steep or long hills where truck engines will be under great strain.)

Poisoned water supplies, dangerous prescription drugs and the over use of X rays have also contributed to the incidence of cancer.

With immune systems constantly battered by polluted air, adulterated and chemically impregnated food and a constant onslaught from the drugs we buy for ourselves, or allow our doctors to prescribe for us, it is not surprising that increasing numbers of people succumb to one of the many different types of cancer. Eight out of ten people who develop cancer could have been saved if money and effort had been put into prevention.

I seriously believe that if I had the annual income the cancer industry enjoys I could turn cancer into a relatively minor disease within five years. (I would also annoy a lot of big industries and most of the medical establishment but I could live with that.)

## The suppression of cures

Cancer is the major league killer of our age and despite the expenditure of billions of dollars and an enormous amount of effort it is getting commoner every year.

However, the medical establishment – operating on behalf of the international pharmaceutical industry and the international food industry – and working with the support of politicians, has deliberately hidden the truth about how cancer is caused. And possible cancer cures have been deliberately suppressed.

The most repressive, most prejudiced, most obscenely intolerant and most ruthlessly dishonest branch of the international medical industry is undoubtedly that part of it which claims to deal with cancer.

Doctors and politicians have cold-bloodedly sacrificed the lives of hundreds of thousands of innocent people solely to protect the interests of a number of major industries.

When a government puts the wealth of a minority above the health of the majority it is fair to conclude that the government is no longer of the people or for the people but has abdicated all responsibility and forfeited the right to respect. Similarly, the medical establishment has forfeited the right to public trust.

## The cancer industry

The cancer industry is now so huge that it requires vast amounts of money simply in order to stay alive. Since a good deal of that money comes from the drug industry (which is, not surprisingly, only interested in pharmacological solutions) the cancer industry's aims, methods and motives are now indistinguishable from the drug industry's aims, methods and motives. Around the world the drug industry has so much control over many cancer charities (because it gives them money) that those cancer charities seem to me to be unhealthily interested in research that is likely to uncover drug based cures. (How could a drug company ever make money out of a treatment programme that involved meditation or a change in diet?)

In addition to being the most intolerant, the modern cancer industry must surely be the least successful branch of medical science ever to have existed. (In my view it is also probably the most corrupt and self-serving. If the cancer industry ever accidentally hit upon a cure for cancer I honestly very much doubt if anyone would hear about it, for finding and publicising a cure for cancer would put the cancer industry employees out of business.)

In order to ensure that money continues to pour in the cancer industry must persuade potential contributors and supporters that it is making progress in the fight against cancer.

But despite the expenditure of billions of dollars on research the cancer industry has consistently and reliably failed to find any answers. Indeed, as has been well documented, the incidence of cancer has been steadily increasing for decades. Chemotherapy does not work and has never worked for the cancers which kill nine out of ten cancer patients. Many patients given chemotherapy and classified as 'cured' go on to develop another cancer within a short period. The cancer establishment has insisted on sticking with radiotherapy and chemotherapy despite the fact that there is much evidence that these approaches do not work. Today, even ordinary patients who have no idea that there are alternatives are turning them down; preferring to die quietly and in peace rather than to die of a painful and pointless treatment programme.

The real problem for the cancer industry is that the enemy isn't just invisible – it simply doesn't exist in the same way that smallpox, tuberculosis or influenza exist. The real problem, the real enemy which has to be confronted, is not a bunch of malignant cells but a weakened, toxin infiltrated body. And since cancer develops when a body is ill and weak it seems pretty obvious to me that the very last thing the body needs when it is ill is to be attacked with toxic chemicals.

(Ironically, the same huge multinational corporations which produce the toxic chemicals which weaken and damage the body and cause cancer to develop also sell the toxic chemicals which are prescribed as a 'cure'. This is the ultimate, exclusively self-serving perpetual motion money machine.)

In America around $110 billion a year is spent on cancer research and treatment. That is more than ten per cent of American's entire health care bill. But, in America, during the last fifteen years or so, the incidence of cancer has steadily risen as has the number of people dying of cancer.

Writing in the European Medical Journal Dr Jack Tropp pointed out that: 'despite the billions of dollars spent each year for cancer research and treatment, using the traditional methods of choice: surgery, chemotherapy and radiation therapy, in the overall picture nothing has changed in the mortality rates in the last thirty five years.'

The only people who benefit from the modern cancer industry are doctors, drug companies and the people who make radiotherapy equipment.

The effort, the money, and all the misguided hope and faith that has been poured into cancer research by the international cancer industry simply hasn't worked.

The cancer industry has failed because it has (in my opinion) deliberately and cold-bloodedly concentrated its efforts on the wrong targets.

## 'Alternative' cancer treatments

One of the great ironies of the our age is the fact that for years now cancer treatments which might work have been made illegal.

Throughout the world, politicians have made sure that the modern cancer industry is protected by law. Bizarrely, in most western countries it is now actually illegal to offer a treatment for cancer that stands a chance of working. Even qualified doctors are only allowed to prescribe chemotherapy or radiotherapy or to send their patients for surgery – despite the fact that the evidence shows that these treatments frequently do more harm than good.

The authorities relentlessly persecute those who offer new and possibly effective and non toxic therapies (ignoring the wishes of patients who want to try those therapies) while condoning, paying for and protecting by law therapies which are known to be often toxic and frequently ineffective.

It is bizarre to see the way that governments tell their citizens that vaccines are all safe, that beef is safe to eat and that chemotherapy is the treatment of choice for cancer.

Doctors who dare to offer patients new hope and new treatments are scorned, abused, persecuted, vilified, forced to go into hiding or threatened with imprisonment.

I could fill pages with the names of honest, caring doctors whose work with cancer patients has won them many followers among the sick and their relatives but has earned them nothing but trouble from the authorities.

The problems faced by the proponents of remedies not made by drug companies have been well documented. Anyone who dares to offer an unofficial remedy for cancer is accused of being simply out to make money. Curiously, this accusation is never made about doctors or drug companies.

In Britain it is illegal for anyone to claim to have a cure for cancer that is not approved by the medical establishment and the pharmaceutical industry. In the US countless cancer pioneers –

including some of the brightest medical brains of the century – have been hounded out of the country and forced to open clinics elsewhere.

There are now many alternative therapies available for the treatment of cancer. Some are available very cheaply. Some are extremely expensive. Some are simple to follow. Some are extremely complex. But the one thing that the successful 'alternative' anti-cancer therapies all have in common is that they improve the health and vitality of the body's immune system and help eradicate chemical toxins from the body.

It seems to me that alternative cancer therapies which work invariably offer diets which are rich in vitamin-packed organic fruit and vegetables and low in toxic chemicals. They also encourage patients to learn how to relax and to find some peace in their lives. It doesn't matter whether the peace comes through meditation, relaxation, religion or love and comfort supplied by people who care.

Those are the stable, ever present qualities of the effective anti-cancer cures which work.

The coffee enemas, the hormone injections and the obscure herbal additions may, in my considered view, be little more than bits of fine tuning which may or may not have an additional healing effect. There is some evidence suggesting that herbal remedies do contain substances which have effective anti-cancer properties but I believe that it is the immune system which is the real key to cancer treatment. I believe that the real benefit from these alternative approaches to cancer comes from the boost the immune system gets from the absence of stress and the high natural vitamin content of the largely fruit and vegetable diet.

With the wholehearted support of politicians being given to the cancer industry, rather than to the welfare of the people who put them in office, the war against cancer will continue to fail. Avoidable cancers will continue to become commoner and commoner and the establishment will continue to ensure that only the toxic (but highly profitable) alleged treatments of cancer which are produced by the pharmaceutical industry will be authorised by governments.

## The 'magic bullet' cure

The cancer industry will not find the all powerful magic bullet cure for which it has been searching now for decades.

It will fail because it is wedded to an interventionist paradigm which depends upon treating the body as a battlefield and the disease as an enemy, and which is modelled upon the way that medicine was practised at the start of the twentieth century when the diseases which worried doctors most were those which were caused by infections – tuberculosis, smallpox, influenza, pneumonia, syphilis, cholera, typhoid fever and so on.

The incidence of these diseases was to a certain extent controlled at the end of the 19th century, and the beginning of the 20th century, and as a result the medical profession as a whole made two crucial and fundamental mistakes.

The first mistake was a retrospective one: it was to assume that the reduction in death rate from these diseases was a result of things which doctors had done. This was quite wrong. The reduction in the incidence of infectious diseases (and, more importantly, the reduction in the number of deaths from those diseases) was a result of better water supplies, better sewage facilities, better transport and better food. The man who invented the water closet saved far more lives than any dozen members of the medical establishment. Mortality rates from infectious diseases had fallen long before the introduction of vaccines and antibiotics (the two remedies favoured by the medical establishment). I will show later in this book that life expectancy for adults has not risen much, if at all, in recent decades or even centuries. Any improvement which has been made has been a result of better living conditions rather than better medicine.

The second fundamental mistake was a prospective one: it was to assume that the interventionist 'magic bullet' approach which appeared to have worked in the war against infectious disease would enable doctors to tackle all other health and life threatening diseases – including cancer. This was a pretty daft mistake to make because most modern killer diseases develop in a very different way to infectious diseases. People get heart disease because they eat too much of the wrong sort of food and not enough of the right sort of food, and because they take too little exercise. And people get cancer because they eat too much of the wrong sort of food and not enough of the right sort of food and because their bodies have been contaminated by toxic, carcinogenic chemicals.

One might have thought that some of the brighter members of the medical establishment might have realised that since modern killer diseases are plainly different to the infectious diseases it might be necessary to think up a different type of treatment approach. But that hasn't happened yet.

And it is this error (no doubt encouraged and compounded by the affection of the medical profession for the money so generously distributed by the pharmaceutical industry) which has led researchers (and doctors) to experiment with increasingly toxic drugs in order to try and 'kill' cancer.

## Chemotherapy

Chemotherapy has repeatedly failed. The medical profession, the pharmaceutical industry and the cancer industry are so desperate to hide this fact that they now probably consider it a success if the survival rate of patients who take chemotherapy actually matches the survival rate of patients who don't take chemotherapy.

There are two fundamental problems with chemotherapy.

First, in order to kill the cancer cells (which are, after all, merely ordinary human cells which have got out of control) the drug which is prescribed must be so toxic that it inevitably causes a great deal of damage to other, healthy, cells. When chemotherapy is given by mouth (or by any other general, system route) the whole body may be affected – even though the drug is aimed only at one very specific site in the body.

When chemotherapy fails to work the doctors invariably respond by increasing the dose or making the chemotherapy even more toxic. The end result is that the chemotherapy may well kill the cancer cells but it will probably also kill the patient. (Thereby helping to perpetuate the old medical comment about the treatment being a success but the patient dying.)

Second, even when chemotherapy (or radiotherapy) does succeed in apparently 'killing' a cancer (and doctors like to give themselves a decent chance at a good cure rate by claiming that any patient who survives an extremely modest five years has been cured) there is a considerable risk that the cancer will recur. When you stop and think about it this isn't difficult to understand for chemotherapy (or radiotherapy or surgery for that matter) does absolutely nothing to alter the circumstances which led to the cancer developing in the first place.

When a cancer recurs it isn't necessarily because the surgeon, the radiotherapist or the physician prescribing the chemotherapy has failed to kill all the cancer cells, but because nothing in the body has changed. The circumstances which led to the development of a first cancer can just as easily lead to the development of a second cancer.

It is for this reason that one often hears of extremely unfortunate individuals who have developed two or even three cancers in separate organs.

However, here's an interesting observation which I bet you won't see plastered all over the official medical journals: twenty years ago when a group of leukaemia patients were treated by having their own bone marrow removed and replaced with bone marrow from a donor, the leukaemia returned in a number of the patients. But – and this is the fascinating bit of the story – DNA checks showed that the new, second bout of leukaemia, consisted of cells which had belonged to the healthy donor. The patient's original bone marrow had all been removed and this time it was the donor's bone marrow which had turned into leukaemia cells.

It seems to me pretty clear from this that there must have been something within those patients' bodies which was turning healthy cells into cancer cells.

And the simple answer is that the cause of the cancer is inside the patient and is untouched by a treatment which simply attacks the cancer cells. It is because the cancer industry either fails to understand this (or doesn't want to believe it) that the cancer industry will never succeed in beating cancer.

All those billions of dollars being pumped into cancer research are being wasted because scientists and doctors insist on attacking an enemy they cannot see and do not understand.

## The underlying cause of cancer

I believe that cancer often develops because the body is weakened and badly damaged. (Although the owner of the body may not be aware of this. Many people who have been under stress and over-exposed to toxins for long periods succeed in suppressing and ignoring the physical and mental signs of distress. They don't feel 'well' but they don't feel 'ill' either – until, one day, a lump is found or an unmistakeable symptom of cancer appears.)

Because of the accumulated stresses, the immune system doesn't work properly and so the toxic chemicals and other irritants which have collected in the body trigger off the development of a cancer.

Where do the toxins and irritants come from?

There is pretty convincing evidence showing that tobacco and toxin-contaminated food (particularly meat) are by far the two biggest causes of cancer. (It is, I believe, because they eat more than their fair share of contaminated food and have toxin-rich fat deposits that overweight individuals are more prone to cancer). Other possible irritants include radiation, polluted air and water, alcohol, drugs, toxins in household and industrial chemicals and electrical fields.

If you don't want to get cancer – or you have cancer and you want to get rid of it – then I believe that the answer is clear: you must reduce your intake of and exposure to toxins and build up your immune system so that it can work harder to defend your body. With an immune system working well you will be less likely to develop cancer.

And if you develop cancer then it is my belief that your body will be better able to destroy the cancer if you improve the efficiency of your immune system and reduce your exposure to toxins.

The importance and vulnerability of the body's immune system cannot be exaggerated. I believe that it is because they overwork their bodies and damage their immune systems that many top international athletes often suffer so much from illness – and tend to die earlier than non athletes. There is a huge difference between fitness and good health.

Sadly, I rather doubt if the medical establishment will ever support this approach for it is an approach to cancer which offers little or nothing in the way of profit to the shareholders and employees of large international companies.

And our existing sad and ineffectual politicians, beholden to big business, will continue to support the cancer industry and for the foreseeable future the official answer to cancer is likely to remain the same as it is at the moment: blast the body with toxic chemicals in the hope that these will kill the cancer tissue. Ironically, the medical establishment, committed as it is to supporting the pharmaceutical industry and the cancer industry, seems unlikely or unwilling to recognise that the other effect of this approach is to damage the immune system, weaken the body and make the organs and tissues within the body more vulnerable not only to the existing cancer but to the development of new cancers too.

## How governments promote cancer

It isn't just the drug industry and the cancer industry which the politicians are trying to protect by denying and suppressing the truth about how cancer develops.

Astonishingly, politicians have also shown themselves to be keen to protect the industries which are known to cause cancer. Of these the two most obvious are the tobacco and food industries.

Despite the fact that the link between tobacco and cancer has been well established for many years politicians have protected and subsidised the tobacco industry for a considerable time. Modern politicians seem to have absolutely no sense of shame. For them hypocrisy is a way of life. Although European governments force tobacco companies to publish health warnings on cigarette packs and advertisements they still give massive subsidies to tobacco farmers. And the Labour government of the late 1990s fought hard to enable tobacco companies to continue promoting their products.

Those of us who prefer to study the evidence and make our own judgements about health issues, rather than listen to and take advice from the various facets of the industry controlled medical and health care establishment, were entitled to feel well justified when the British government at long last looked to be about to warn its citizens that the consumption of meat is linked to the development of cancer.

But after considering the (incontrovertible) evidence for some months Britain's much welcomed Labour government responded instead to a warning from the meat industry that publishing the truth about the link between meat and cancer would result in lost jobs and a blow to the economy. The financial threat was enough to end the possibility of the government publicising the truth about the link between meat and cancer.

Politicians have actually gone further than simply refusing to publicise the true facts about meat and cancer – they (and other members of the establishment) have done everything they can to suppress the truth – purely because of the fear that the truth might damage the meat industry.

I have repeatedly warned readers that eating meat can lead to the development of cancers of the breast, colon, prostate, endometrium (lining of the uterus), rectum, pancreas and kidney (see my book *Power Over Cancer*, published by the European Medical Journal for the evidence) but to their eternal shame, politicians, doctors and bureaucrats still insist on ignoring the evidence – and protecting the meat industry.

## 10. The Danger Of Electromagnetic Fields

There are many ways in which our modern environment can cause cancer, can damage the human immune system and can increase our susceptibility and vulnerability to many different types of disease – including infections and cancer.

But electricity is almost certainly a much bigger cause of problems – and far more dangerous – than most people imagine.

73

If you spend most of your time working with or close to an electrical appliance, if you live or work near to an electricity supply line or if you spend your days working with electrical equipment then the chances of you developing cancer of one sort or another are considerably increased.

Of course, the men in suits won't tell you this. They'll frighten you half to death about minority threats such as AIDS and radon because the former is a politically and commercially useful threat and the latter seems like an excellent way to boost the building industry, but they won't give you any warning about the danger of electricity because they don't want to annoy the many large and powerful business interests which sell, market, service or supply electricity and electrical equipment.

I certainly think that the evidence is pretty convincing. And in America, where people only vote with their wallets when they really believe something, house prices near to electricity supply lines have fallen dramatically in recent years.

Just look at these facts:

- The dean of a school of public health has said: 'The present state of affairs is like the correlation between smoking and lung cancer 30 years ago'. He added that, at a conservative estimate, a third of all childhood cancers are caused by electrical fields.

- A study of nearly 500 children showed that children whose mothers used electric blankets when they were pregnant were two and a half times as likely to develop brain tumours.

- A study of nearly 700 children showed that children who lived in houses near to power distribution lines were two or three times as likely to die of leukaemia or brain tumours.

- A study at an American University showed that men who work as electricians or electrical engineers are ten times as likely to develop certain types of brain tumour.

- Experts found that workers for a telephone company who worked alongside electricity power lines were seven times as likely to develop leukaemia.

In my view the threat doesn't just come from power lines –

any electromagnetic field can be a danger. The closer you are to an electrical or magnetic field – the greater the danger.

The industry experts don't agree with me about these hazards. They insist that electricity is safe. But would they tell you if they thought it wasn't? And can you trust them?

In my view there is ample evidence to show that people who spend too much time close to electrical appliances (and, in particular, to power lines) are more likely to develop cancer. Not that cancer is the only possible hazard associated with electricity. Severe and persistent headaches, muscle pain, otherwise unexplained fatigue, damaged immune system (with a resultant increased susceptibility to infection as well as cancer), Parkinson's disease, Alzheimer's disease, multiple sclerosis, chronic fatigue syndrome (myalgic encephalomyelitis), cataracts and pregnancy problems are some of the other possible dangers which may be linked to exposure to electromagnetic fields and radiation.

While writing this book I received information that the American government has suppressed research work which took nine years to complete and which verified the link between electrosmog (electromagnetic fields), cerebral illnesses and cancer.

The suppressed report was compiled for the US government and I am informed that it concludes: 'Even weak electromagnetic fields can impair health.... They lead to disturbance of the production of the hormone melatonin, which is known to be an important biochemical link. A deficit in this hormone favours the developing of, for example, breast cancer as well as the developing of degenerative cerebral illnesses such as Parkinson's disease or Alzheimer's disease, but also brings on heart problems.'

The suppressed report also confirms that electromagnetic fields can bring on leukaemia in children.

'In addition,' continue the authors of the report, 'there is an increased risk of developing leukaemia and also brain tumours for adults who are exposed to strong fields due to their professions.'

The assumption is that the electromagnetic fields cause a disturbance in the biochemical function of the cells, or influence certain genes. Both mechanisms can cause permanent damage to the cells. (Genetic engineers use electromagnetic radiation to open cell membranes and insert alien genes.

The authors of this suppressed report also point out that interactions between electromagnetic rays and the cells of the immune system can favour the beginning of cancer – and that the influence of electromagnetic fields on the reproductive organs may cause disease there too.

The authors of this suppressed study demand that more research be done and that threshold values for the intensity of electromagnetic fields be lowered to a level that would be exceeded by modern electrical wiring and ordinary household appliances.

The study also suggests that overhead power lines may be a significant threat to human health. The threshold values recommended by this suppressed US report are 5000 times lower than the internationally recognised threshold values.

It is not difficult to see why the US government has suppressed this report. If the findings of the report were implemented vast industries would be affected and very few factories, offices or homes would be considered safe.

As an interim measure the authors of this study demand that what they call the 'permanent radiation bombardment' to which we are all subjected should be reduced step by step. They recommend that all overhead power lines should be removed from residential areas and that houses and schools should no longer be built anywhere near to power lines.

Sadly, I am less surprised by the fact that this report was suppressed than I would have been if it had been published. Modern politicians are controlled by big companies and their lobbyists.

## Mobile phones and transmitters

Mobile telephones are a fast developing major source of hazardous electromagnetic fields.

Mobile telephones use microwave radiation to transmit conversations between handsets and base-stations and between base-stations and handsets.

The early (and most obvious fear) was that using a mobile telephone while driving, or performing any other intricate and potential hazardous activity, would inevitably increase any individual's chances of having an accident.

However, since the early 1980s, when mobile telephones first became popular, there have been worries about the possible damage that these microwaves could do to the human brain. Some experts have suggested that using one of these telephones could create short term memory loss while others have argued that they could cause brain tumours.

When mobile phones were bulky, extremely expensive and scarce no one worried much about these fears. But today the number of people using mobile telephones is increasing dramatically.

This rapid increase in the number of people using mobile phones means that governments and health authorities have to pretend to take notice (although if the commercial opposition to action is powerful enough the discovery of worrying information will not necessarily mean that they will do anything). If mobile phones prove to be as hazardous to health as some people say they could be the implications for government health care expenditure could be awesome.

Insurance companies are never slow to take notice of new health risks. It may, therefore, be of some significance that one of the world's largest insurance companies is now reported to be including a clause in its personal liability policies which excludes: 'Damage to persons caused by electromagnetic fields'.

When thousands of people used mobile telephones a small increase in the chances of developing a brain tumour would only result in a tiny increase in the overall incidence of brain cancer. However, now that millions use mobile telephones the same modest risk could result in a huge rise in the number of people requiring attention for serious health problems. Studies have shown that 20-80% of the electromagnetic radiation generated by mobile telephones is absorbed directly into the user's brain. (The rest of the radiation goes in other directions and can affect other human beings nearby.) Just a few minutes' exposure to cell phone radiation can turn a 5% active cancer into a 95% active cancer.

Several research groups have begun studies to find out if

there really is a link between the long term use of mobile telephones and the incidence of brain tumours.

But at the moment the short answer to the questions about this hazard is that no one really seems to know what the risks are.

In America there have (inevitably perhaps) already been a number of lawsuits brought by mobile telephone users who have developed brain tumours. The number of lawsuits is rising. As far as I am aware none of these lawsuits have been successful though doctors have observed that when mobile phone users develop brain cancers the cancer tends to be behind the ear against which the telephone is habitually held. (So, if you prefer a left sided brain tumour hold your mobile telephone against your left ear).

Lawyers defending mobile phone companies will undoubtedly argue that all this is just a coincidence but in Australia an oncologist has suggested that a 50% increase in the incidence of brain tumours in Western Australia between 1982 and 1992 could have been caused by the increase in the use of mobile telephones during that period. You will, I know, be surprised to hear that there does not seem to be a great deal of support within the mobile telephone industry for this point of view.

In theory I don't think there is much doubt that the sort of microwaves used by mobile telephones could harm the brain. In Denmark scientists have expressed surprise that people who would (presumably) be reluctant to put their heads into a microwave oven are happy to 'cook' their brains by holding a mobile telephone to the side of their head for hours on end. Like other forms of electromagnetic radiation mobile telephones can induce electrical currents and they can make body tissues hotter. There is a real possibility that these effects could disrupt electrical activity within brain cells – or even damage DNA.

In one way the risks associated with mobile telephones are relatively slight. A mobile phone produces only around 1 watt of energy – a great deal less than a microwave oven which will probably produce around 600 watts.

But, on the other hand, the big problem is that mobile telephones are, inevitably, held close to the brain while being used. Not many people stand holding microwave ovens next to their brains for minutes at a time! Worse still is the fact that the mobile telephone is likely to be held in pretty much the same position every time it is used – with the same portion of brain being affected. And, of course, some people seem to spend hours talking on their mobile telephones.

Whatever the risks associated with mobile telephones may be, the risks associated with the base transmitting stations (which are essential for the functioning of the mobile telephone service) may be considerably greater for those individuals who live close by.

Base stations continually irradiate those living, working and studying nearby and although the doses of radiation are much lower than the doses produced by portable telephones or microwave ovens there may be a serious health risk. I just don't think anyone really knows just how great that risk may be – or whether it is greater or smaller than the risk associated with overhead power lines. Given the option I would prefer not to live next to a mobile telephone base station just as I would prefer not to live under a power line.

How far away is safe? I can't tell you and I don't think anyone else can either. I certainly wouldn't want to be nearer than 150 yards to a transmitter.

Up until recently there has been very little evidence available to show that transmitters can be dangerous. However, a good deal of work has been done in Switzerland in the last couple of years. For example, researchers have shown that trees have been severely damaged by mobile phone transmitter masts.

And in Schwarzenburg, Switzerland protestors recently managed to close down an international radio station.

After complaints from the public 200 people living in the irradiated area were compared with 200 people in a radiation free zone in order to find out whether the transmitter did have an effect on the health of local individuals.

The study showed that serious sleep disorders were five times as common among individuals living in the irradiated area; that depressions were four times as common; that cancer was three times as common and that diabetes was twice as common. Interestingly, these disorders occurred in areas where the electromagnetic field intensity was much lower than the official accepted safety level.

(Official safety levels do not seem to be high. Indeed, the safety levels in some countries seems to have been set at a point that will enable companies to put antenna masts right in the heart of residential areas and alongside schools and hospitals.)

The results of the study in Schwarzenburg were so alarming that the authorities took action and the transmitter was taken down.

When the transmitter had been demolished numerous residents stated that they were sleeping better and that pains in joints and limbs had all but disappeared. Depressed residents said that they felt better and overactive children became much quieter.

We still don't know the health risks involved with using a mobile phone and we don't know yet whether long term use will increase your chances of developing brain cancer. I would like to see a good deal more research being done to investigate a health hazard which affects vast numbers of people. However, official money is unlikely to be available to investigate a potential problem which could threaten one of the world's fastest growing industries.

As I was preparing this book I learned that the Australian government was giving researchers £500,000 to expose genetically engineered mice to radio waves from mobile phones. Allegedly, this was being done to 'study the possible dangers to human users'. I wrote an article forecasting that if the results show that the mice were undamaged by the radio waves the research might be hailed as proof that phones are safe for human use, whereas if the results showed that the mice developed cancer the research might be dismissed on the grounds that animals are different to people. (This is the technique which was used for years by the tobacco industry when animals were forced to smoke cigarettes. The same double-edged trick is also commonly used by the drug industry.)

After hearing about the proposed Australian research I learned that experiments on genetically engineered mice had already shown that mice who are exposed to cell phone radiation are twice as likely to develop lymphoma (a type of cancer).

And, as predicted, this evidence had been dismissed as irrelevant on the grounds that results obtained from experiments on animals cannot be applied to human beings.

The mobile phone industry is now one of the fastest growing and most profitable industries in the world. My cynical but honest (and, I fear, accurate) prediction is that whatever evidence is unearthed no research establishing a firm link between mobile telephones and brain cancer will be officially recognised and accepted for at least two decades – if ever.

Incidentally, in 1999 a report was published claiming that people who use mobile telephones had faster reaction times. Some users of mobile telephones leapt upon this report as evidence that mobile phones must be safe to use. However, this research found a very modest (4%) improvement in reaction times among people who had used an (artificial) mobile phone for half an hour. It is possible that the slight improvement in reaction time might have been due to the heating effect of the microwaves – possibly because the heating speeded up some chemical reaction in the brain or stimulated blood flow. In my view, this research certainly doesn't prove that mobile telephones are safe. My serious fear about mobile phones is that long term exposure may cause brain damage.

# Part Three: How You Can Strengthen Your Immune System And Protect Yourself From Infections And Cancer

In this, the final part of *Superbody*, I will explain how you can reduce your exposure to cancer and infectious disease and how you can strengthen your body's immune system – and keep it in tip top condition – so that you will be better able to survive in the 21st century.

## 1. Eat Foods That Will Boost Your Immune System

Your body's immune system helps to protect you against infection. If your immune system – your inbuilt defence system – is in tip-top condition then you will be far less vulnerable to marauding viruses or bacteria. Your body will also be better able to fight cancer – and win. What you choose to eat can have a big effect on the strength and effectiveness of your immune system.

Most people know what foods they shouldn't eat. They understand that if they live on a diet of hamburgers and chips, followed by chocolate pudding covered with lashings of double cream, and all washed down with a cola drink, then their health will suffer.

If you eat meat it is important that you give it up – particularly if you have an infection which is being treated with antibiotics – or eat only organically grown meat. The spread of a number of killer infections has been traced to meat shipments. The basic cause is simple: farmers routinely feed antibiotics to their animals to keep them healthy. Animals which are fed with antibiotics inevitably acquire antibiotic resistant organisms. Repeated problems caused by meat infected with antibiotic-resistant bugs are a direct result of this still unregulated and uncontrolled farming practice.

Many of the people who fall ill after eating infected meat have been taking antibiotics – for throat or ear infections for example. The antibiotic prescribed for the throat or ear infection clears the body of many of its natural infections, allowing the antibiotic-resistant superbug to take over a virtually competitor - free body.

If you eat eggs do not ever buy (or eat) eggs with cracked shells. It is much easier for an infection to enter an egg with a cracked shell. Eggs laid by genuinely free range chickens are likely to be healthier than eggs laid by hens kept in battery cages.

Finding out exactly what you should eat isn't quite so easy. The truth is shrouded in mystery and confusion – much of created, quite deliberately, on behalf of vested interests, by lobbyists, advertising agencies and public relations groups.

The far reaching tentacles of the big food companies are as powerful as those of the big drug companies. Finding the truth is made particularly difficult by the fact that many newspapers, magazines and journals readily publish material they are given by companies with products to sell. Television and radio are, of course, just as likely to publicise these commercial messages disguised as independent news items.

Frequently, undue emphasis is placed on small – often almost irrelevant bits and pieces of scientific information – which are fed to the media because they help to build up and strengthen some hidden agenda. Too many observers (by which I mean editors, journalists and commentators) fail to analyse the information which appears; seemingly ignorant of the fact that an overview is necessary if any information is going to be put into perspective and used effectively.

Hyperbole and exaggeration used to be the preserve of the tabloid newspapers. These days they are everyday tools for broadsheet journalists and for just about everyone working in television and radio.

Sponsorship is widespread and often subtle, and this can make it difficult to decide exactly what is true and what isn't. Hidden agendas are sometimes well hidden, sometimes hidden only a little and sometimes not hidden at all.

I have prepared a list of the 101 healthiest, tastiest and very best foods in the world. These are foods that don't just taste good and look good – they will provide you with a massive amount of protection against cancer and heart disease, they will boost your immune system and they help reduce your susceptibility to infection.

And whether they agree or disagree with the contents of this list you can be confident that no one has sponsored this list.

Naturally, you don't have to limit yourself to the foods on this list which I have compiled as a starting point: a healthy basis for any good, well-balanced, diet.

The list will, I hope, also help the many readers who have written to me explaining that they plan to become vegetarian (or vegan) but confessing that they really don't know what to eat.

I've arranged this list in alphabetical order – partly because I think it will make it easier to use, and partly because I didn't want to print a list that suggested that any one particular food was 'number one'!

To make the list more accessible I haven't listed all the specific nutrients and health giving ingredients these foods contain but have simply given a very brief summary of the main qualities of individual foods.

Foods which contain antioxidants (such as vitamins C and E, the mineral selenium and beta-carotene, which is converted in the human body to vitamin A) help prevent cancer and heart disease and reduce susceptibility to infection.

My recommended healthy diet would contain a good and varied selection of foods from this list.

### 1. Alfalfa sprouts
Low in protein and don't contain much in the way of minerals or vitamins but they are also low in fat, calories and sodium. They are a tasty filler for salads and sandwiches.

### 2. Almonds
Rich in vitamin E (an antioxidant), plus calcium and protein. (But watch out: they also contain a high proportion of fat.)

### 3. Apple
Contain antioxidants. Will help strengthen your immune system. Plenty of fibre and vitamin C.

### 4. Apricots
Like all orange-coloured fruits and vegetables apricots are packed with the antioxidant beta-carotene which helps protect against cancer. Apricots are also full of fibre. Dried apricots make an excellent snack food. (Buy organic dried apricots not the bright orange ones).

### 5. Artichoke
May help reduce blood fat and cholesterol levels and may help with liver, gall bladder and digestive problems.

### 6. Asparagus
Has a diuretic effect and is also believed to be useful in the treatment of nausea, heartburn and hiatus hernia.

### 7. Aubergine (eggplant)
In South East Asia some people use it to treat stomach cancer. Not a food to fry because it absorbs huge amounts of fat.

### 8. Avocado pear
Technically a berry rather than a pear. Contains 14 minerals, 11 vitamins and plenty of protein. Low in sodium. May contain special anti bacterial and anti fungal ingredients. Some say the avocado has anti-cancer properties.

### 9. Baked beans
Excellent source of fibre.

### 10. Bananas
Packed with vitamins, minerals, fibre and carbohydrate and low in fat. Excellent source of potassium.

### 11. Bean sprouts
A good source of vitamins B and C. Also contain protein.

### 12. Beans
A good source of potassium and folate. May help prevent or treat anaemia. May help reduce the risk of heart disease. High in fibre and protein. Pulses are usually low in fat.

### 13. Beetroot
Good source of folate and iron.

### 14. Bilberry (a.k.a. blueberry)
Believed to help improve the circulation and to counteract urinary tract infections. Bilberries have antioxidant, anti-inflammatory and anti infective effects.

### 15. Blackberries
Excellent low fat source of vitamin E.

### 16. Blackcurrant
An excellent source of vitamin C. (Weight for weight blackcurrants contain four times as much vitamin C as oranges). Moreover the blackcurrant retains its vitamin C content well. Blackcurrants contain anthocyanins which are anti-inflammatory and which inhibit bacteria such as E.coli, holidaying merrily among the villae of the intestinal riviera.

### 17. Bread
Wholemeal bread is rich in fibre and vitamins and minerals.

### 18. Broad beans
A good source of protein and soluble fibre.

### 19. Broccoli
Contain antioxidants and other substances which provide protection against cancer. Cancers which may be prevented – or slowed – by broccoli, cauliflower, cabbage and brussels sprouts include cancer of the breast, cancer of the colon and stomach cancer. Most useful when eaten raw. Overcooking dramatically reduces its value.

### 20. Brussels sprouts
Contain antioxidants and other substances which provide protection against cancer.

### 21. Cabbage
Contains substances which provide protection against cancer.

### 22. Carrot
Contain antioxidants. Full of fibre, vitamins and minerals. A great, healthy snack food. I often stuff a carrot and an apple in my bag when travelling.

### 23. Cauliflower
Contain antioxidants and other substances which provide protection against cancer.

### 24. Celeriac
A good source of potassium. When eaten raw (e.g. in salads) it is also a good source of vitamin C.

### 25. Celery
Nearly calorie free but nevertheless nutritious.

### 26. Cherries
Contain potassium and vitamin C.

### 27. Chestnuts
High in carbohydrates and fibre but, unusually for nuts, low in fat. Brazil nuts, walnuts and hazelnuts have more than twenty times as much fat as chestnuts. Contain vitamin E and vitamin B6.

### 28. Chickpeas
Will help reduce cholesterol levels. Impecunious Indians who live on a chickpea diet have low blood cholesterol. Contain antioxidants.

### 29. Chillies
Chilli pepper may help desensitise the airways and may help stop an asthma attack. By having a mildly irritant effect on the stomach chillies may also stimulate the stomach to defend itself against more serious threats – and may help to protect against damage and the development of ulcers. The substance which gives chillies their fierce flavour is capsaicin which is an antioxidant which helps provide protection against cancer.

### 30. Corn
Contains protein, iron, zinc and potassium. Low in sodium. The Tarahumara Indians of Mexico live on a diet of corn and beans.

High blood cholesterol and artery clogging and their fateful consequences are virtually unknown among these people. Contain antioxidants.

### 31. Courgettes (Zucchini)
A type of small marrow and a useful source of vitamin C and folate. Also a good source of beta-carotene. Most of the nutrients are stored in the skins, which are edible.

### 32. Cranberry
Widely used as a home remedy in the treatment of bladder, kidney and urinary tract infection. It used to be thought that this was because cranberries have a high acid content but recent research has shown that cranberries contain something which prevents infectious bacteria from multiplying in the urinary tract. The only other fruit to have a similar effect is the bilberry (a.k.a. blueberry).

### 33. Cress
A cruciferous vegetable which can help prevent the development of cancer. Rich in vitamins and minerals. May help prevent anaemia and heart disease.

### 34. Dates
Dried dates are rich in potassium and a good source of many other nutrients too (including iron). A nourishing source of sugar.

### 35. Fennel
Toasted fennel seeds are chewed in India to prevent indigestion and bad breath. Alternatively the seeds can be used to make a tea which helps digestive problems including flatulence and colic. Fennel seeds should be avoided during pregnancy.

### 36. Figs
Rich in potassium and fibre. Also contain pectin which can help lower blood cholesterol levels.

### 37. Garlic
Garlic, onions, chives, leeks and shallots will all provide protection against cancer, infection and heart disease. I believe that garlic can help bring down high blood pressure, lower blood cholesterol levels, help prevent blood clotting and dilate blood vessels. Probably my No 1 'magic' food.

### 38. Ginger
Helps relieve nausea, flatulence and indigestion. May stimulate the circulation and prevent blood clots. May also relieve rheumatism. Ginger keeps many of its properties when dried.

### 39. Grapefruit
Packed with vitamins (especially vitamin C) and rich in fibre. Will help strengthen the immune system. Contains antioxidants. Pink grapefruit contains lycopene which helps provide protection against cancer (particularly prostate cancer) and heart disease.

### 40. Grapes
Grapes contain ellagic acid which may help prevent cancer developing. (Cherries and strawberries contain the same substance).

### 41. Hazel nuts
Contain vitamin E (an antioxidant) plus vitamins B1 and B6. Also contain protein. The downside is a high fat content.

### 42. Hummus
Contains chickpeas, sesame seeds, garlic, coriander seeds, lemon juice and olive oil. It is, consequently, packed with goodness (but buy a low fat version).

### 43. Kale
A very good source of vitamin C and beta-carotene. Also, like other deep green vegetables, kale is a good source of calcium and iron. It also contains compounds which may provide protection against cancer.

### 44. Kidney beans
A good source of protein. Contains potassium, zinc and iron. But be careful: raw or undercooked kidney beans can cause serious food poisoning.

### 45. Lentils
A good source of protein, fibre, minerals and vitamins.

### 46. Lettuce
Lettuce (and other salad greens) provide protection against cancer (particularly cancer of the stomach). Also contains the antioxidant vitamins C and E. A good source of iron. May also aid digestion.

### 47. Lime
May help to reduce cancer risk. May also help to prevent infection. A good source of potassium.

### 48. Linseed
A good source of omega 3 fatty acids which lower the risk of colorectal cancer by reducing the amount of prostaglandin in the bowel. May aid digestion and prevent constipation. May also help prevent breast cancer and may help ease menopausal symptoms.

### 49. Lychees
An excellent source of vitamin C.

### 50. Mango
A useful source of vitamins C and E when raw. Also contain iron. A good source of carotene – particularly when ripe.

### 51. Melon
Water melon contains lycopene which helps provide protection against cancer (particularly prostate cancer) and heart disease. Melon with orange flesh (such as cantaloupe) is rich in carotene.

### 52. Mushrooms
Contain protein, vitamins and minerals but are low in fat and calories. Rich in potassium, iron and niacin. Some varieties may discourage the development of cancer.

### 53. Mustard
Mustard (commonly grown with cress) may help prevent cancer and heart disease.

### 54. Oats
Oat bran contains protein, carbohydrate and vitamin B – and is packed with fibre. Oat bran will help reduce your blood cholesterol level.

### 55. Olive oil
Cold pressed extra virgin olive oil is a good source of vitamin E.

### 56. Olives
A good source of vitamin E.

### 57. Onions
Onions, chives, leeks and shallots may all provide protection against

cancer, infection and heart disease.

## 58. Orange

Contain antioxidants. Packed with vitamins (particularly vitamin C) and rich in fibre.

## 59. Papaya (pawpaw)

Contains carotene and vitamin C and, when raw, an enzyme which digests protein.

## 60. Parsley

Contains protein and useful amounts of vitamins and minerals.

## 61. Parsnip

A useful source of starch and fibre and of vitamins C and E.

## 62. Passion fruit

Contain vitamin C.

## 63. Pasta

Contain lots of complex carbohydrate and fibre and is low in fat.

## 64. Peaches

Rich in vitamin C. Dried peaches contain a good deal of potassium.

## 65. Pears

A good source of natural sugar. Contain some vitamins.

## 66. Peas

Rich in vitamin B1 and a good source of vitamin C. Contain fibre, protein, phosphorus and folate.

## 67. Peppers

An excellent source of vitamin C. Red peppers contain more vitamin C than green peppers and are also an excellent source of beta-carotene.

## 68. Pine nuts

Contain iron, manganese, magnesium and zinc – as well as vitamin B1 and vitamin E (an antioxidant). Also contain protein. Downside is a high fat content.

## 69. Pineapple

Contain antioxidants.

### 70. Pinto beans
High in protein and fibre and low in fat.

### 71. Plums
Contain vitamin E and potassium.

### 72. Pomegranate
A good source of vitamin C.

### 73. Potato
Perhaps the most undervalued food in the world. Rich in vitamins (particularly vitamin C) – especially if eaten in their jackets.

### 74. Prunes
Contain vitamins and minerals as well as heaps of fibre. Good to add to breakfast cereals or salads. Gentle laxative effect.

### 75. Pumpkin
Packed with cancer preventing beta-carotene plus plenty of other vitamins and minerals – and fibre too. Pumpkin seeds, which contain zinc, are widely used to help prevent (and treat) prostate enlargement.

### 76. Radishes
Useful source of vitamin C.

### 77. Raspberries
Rich in vitamin C.

### 78. Redcurrant
Rich in vitamin C and potassium.

### 79. Rhubarb
A good source of potassium.

### 80. Rice
Brown rice contains antioxidants. Rice bran may help reduce the risk of bowel cancer. A good source of starch.

### 81. Runner beans
Contain iron, folate and vitamin C.

### 82. Seaweed
Contains beta-carotene and B vitamins as well as many minerals. Most types of seaweed are a good source of iodine.

### 83. Sesame seeds
Contain vitamin E and calcium.

### 84. Soya beans
Contains antioxidants. Excellent source of protein. Soya milks and yoghurts contain plenty of protein and little sugar. Soya is used in production of textured vegetable protein (TVP) which is (in addition to being a good protein source) an excellent source of zinc, calcium, iron and B vitamins.

### 85. Spinach
Contains antioxidants. Rich in minerals, fibre and protein as well as vitamins. Can be used in salads as well as cooked. (The usual mistake is to overcook it so that it becomes tasteless and of little nutritional value.)

### 86. Squash (Winter)
Pumpkins and other winter squash are a good source of beta-carotene.

### 87. Strawberries
Contains antioxidants. One of the richest sources of vitamin C.

### 88. Sunflower oil
Rich in vitamin E.

### 89. Sunflower seeds
Rich in zinc.

### 90. Swedes
May help to prevent cancer. A good source of vitamin C.

### 91. Sweet Potato (yam)
Contains antioxidants.

### 92. Tea
A gentle stimulant which also supplies an antioxidant which may lower the risk of cancer and heart disease.

### 93. Tomatoes
Contain lycopene which helps provide protection against cancer – particularly prostate cancer. Men who eat tomato based foods (particularly tomato ketchup, canned tomatoes, tomato soup, tomato based spaghetti sauce and the tomato sauce used in prepar-

ing pizza) are less likely to develop prostate cancer. Lycopene may also protect against heart disease and other cancers. It is the heat processing which seems to increase the availability of lycopene in tomatoes. So frying tomatoes should also increase their lycopene availability.

## 94. Turnip
A good source of fibre and vitamin C.

## 95. Walnut
Help lower blood cholesterol and may help prevent heart disease. Rich in essential fatty acids which are vital for tissue growth and development.

## 96. Watercress
Rich in vitamins and minerals but virtually calorie free.

## 97. Wheat
The consumption of wheat fibre is linked to a lower cancer risk (particularly breast cancer). May help relieve menopausal symptoms and prevent heart disease.

## 98. Wheatgerm
The most nutrient rich part of wheat. Provides vitamins B and E.

## 99. Wine
Red wine drinkers seem to have a reduced incidence of heart disease. Moderation is the key. One or two glasses a day seem ideal. Red wine is also believed to have an antioxidant effect (and may provide some protection against viruses too).

## 100. Wholegrains
Wholegrain barley, buckwheat, maize and rye may help prevent heart disease, high blood pressure, diabetes and some cancers.

## 101. Yoghurt
Natural yoghurt is high in calcium and protein and a good source of iron and vitamins in the B group. Most important, perhaps, yoghurt often contains lactobacilli which compete with and oust numerous infections including thrush. Soya yoghurt is also available.

## 2. Cut Your Fat Consumption

If you eat too much cholesterol there is a risk that your body's white cells − crucial warriors in your body's immune system defences − may be damaged. And if you have lots of fat in your blood that will also affect your body's ability to deal with infections.

In a normal, healthy body white cells constantly patrol your blood stream hunting out bacteria (and stray cancer cells). If your blood stream is clogged with fat your white cells simply cannot move around effectively.

Imagine how difficult it would be for a group of lifeguards to swim through an oilslick and you'll have an idea of just how difficult it is for white cells to move through fat soaked blood.

Incidentally, all fats are bad for your immune system but animal fats are probably worse than others, and can probably do more damage to your immune system. One of the reasons for this is the fact that animal fat is often contaminated with chemical residues − toxic and possibly carcinogenic residues of drugs consumed (accidentally or deliberately) by feeding animals.

It is often difficult to find out how much fat there is in particular foods. And it is often terribly easy to eat foods which contain a lot of fat without realising it. This specially produced list below is designed to help solve that problem. It may contain a few surprises!

Remember that the figures on this list are only approximate figures intended to be used as a general guide. And remember that if you cook in additional fat the effective fat content of the food you are cooking will rise − often dramatically!

Governments often recommend that a healthy diet should contain no more than 30% fat. I think that figure is far too high (probably because a relatively high fat diet helps keep the food industry rich and happy). I believe that you should aim to have no more than 15-20% fat in your diet. If for some reason you need to follow a low fat diet you may wish to cut your consumption of fat to 10-15%. (There is more about fat − and other foodstuffs − in my book *Food for Thought*.)

To calculate the percentage of fat in foods which are not on this list look at the calorie list on the package label and divide the number of calories obtained from fat by the total number of calories; then multiply that total by 100 to obtain the percentage.

Almonds 56%
Anchovies 20%
Anchovy, canned, drained 20%
Apple 1%
Apple juice 0%
Apple, baked 0%
Apricot 0%
Artichoke 0%
Asparagus 0%
Aubergine 0%
Avocado pear 22%
Bacon, back fried 44%
Bacon, back grilled 35%
Bacon, streaky 38%
Baked beans 1%
Banana 0%
Beans, green 0%
Beans, kidney 1%
Beans, lentils 0%
Beans, lima 0%
Beans, pinto 0%
Beef, minced 26%
Beef, roast 34%
Beef suet 95%
Beefburger 27%
Beer 0%
Beetroot 0%
Biscuits, chocolate (digestives) 24%
Biscuits, chocolate chip 20%
Biscuits, cream sandwich 26%
Biscuits, digestive 20%
Biscuits, macaroon 23%

Biscuits, plain (rich tea/lincoln) 17%
Black pudding 25%
Blackberries 0%
Blackcurrant drink 0%
Blackcurrants 0%
Bran 6%
Bran flakes 2%
Bran wheat 5%
Brazil nuts 61%
Bread, brown 2%
Bread, Currant 8%
Bread, English muffin 2%
Bread, French stick 3%
Bread, granary 3%
Bread roll (white) 7%
Bread, rye 2%
Bread, soda 3%
Bread, wheatgerm 2%
Bread, white 2%
Bread, white, fried 32%
Bread, white, toasted 1%
Bread, wholemeal 3%
Broad beans 1%
Broccoli 0%
Brown sauce 0%
Brussels sprouts 0%
Butter 82%
Cabbage 0%
Carrot 0%
Cashew nuts, roasted, unsalted 46%
Cauliflower 0%
Caviar, black 16%
Celery 0%
Chapatti 1%
Cheese, Austrian smoked 22%
Cheese, Blue Brie 38%
Cheese, Boursin 42%

Cheese, Brie 27%
Cheese, Caerphilly 31%
Cheese, Camembert 23%
Cheese, Cheddar 33%
Cheese, Cheshire 31%
Cheese, Cottage (low fat) 2%
Cheese, Cream 47%
Cheese, Danish Blue 30%
Cheese, Double Gloucester 34%
Cheese, Edam 28%
Cheese, Emmenthal 30%
Cheese, Feta 20%
Cheese, Fromage Frais 7%
Cheese, Gorgonzola 34%
Cheese, Gouda 31%
Cheese, Gruyere 32%
Cheese, Lancashire 31%
Cheese, Leicester 34%
Cheese, Marscarpone 46%
Cheese, Mozarella 21%
Cheese, Parmesan 33%
Cheese, Roquefort 31%
Cheese, Stilton, blue 35%
Cheese, Stilton, white 31%
Cheese, Wensleydale 31%
Cherries 0%
Chestnuts 3%
Chick-peas 2%
Chicken, dark meat, no skin 6%
Chicken, light meat, no skin 5%
Chicken, roast 14%
Chicory 0%
Chilies 1%
Chinese leaves 0%
Chocolate bar, milk 30%
Chocolate bar, plain 30%
Chocolate bar with nuts 26%

Chocolate drink 6%
Chutney 0%
Cider 0%
Cockles, shelled 1%
Cocoa 20%
Coconut, shredded 35%
Cod, steamed 1%
Cod, grilled 1%
Cod fillet in batter 10%
Cod's roe 4%
Coffee 0%
Cola drink 0%
Coleslaw 5%
Coley, raw 1%
Corn, canned, cream style 1%
Corn, canned 1%
Corn on the cob, fresh 0%
Cornflakes 1%
Corned beef 33%
Courgettes 0%
Crabmeat 5%
Cranberry sauce 0%
Cream, aerosol spray 32%
Cream, clotted 64%
Cream, double 48%
Cream, Fraiche, Half fat 10%
Cream, Fraiche 27%
Cream, half cream 14%
Cream, single 20%
Cream, sour 20%
Cream, whipping 39%
Cream crackers 16%
Crispbread 2%
Crumpet 1%
Cucumber 0%
Custard 4%
Danish pastry 26%

Dates, dried 1%
Duck, roasted without skin 10%
Duck's egg 14%
Egg, boiled 11%
Egg, fried 19%
Egg, omelette 16%
Figs, dried 0%
Figs, fresh 0%
Fish cakes (fried) 11%
Fish fingers (fried) 13%
Fish paste 10%
Flour, white 1%
Flour, wholemeal 2%
Gammon rasher 12%
Garlic 0%
Gin, whisky, vodka, brandy 0%
Ginger ale 0%
Goat's milk 5%
Golden syrup 0%
Goose 22%
Gooseberries 0%
Grapefruit 0%
Grapefruit juice, unsweetened 0%
Grapes, black 0%
Grapes, white 0%
Gravy (meat juices, fat, flour and stock) 9%
Haddock fillet, smoked 1%
Halibut, steamed 16%
Ham 26%
Hazel nuts 36%
Herring, grilled 13%
Herring, pickled 18%
Herring, raw 18%
Herring, rollmop 10%
Honey 0%
Horseradish sauce 8%
Hot dog sausages 25%

Ice cream 16%
Jam 0%
Jelly 0%
Kidney, fried 6%
Kipper, baked 45%
Kipper, grilled 11%
Kiwi fruit 1%
Lager 0%
Lamb chop, grilled 22%
Lamb leg, roasted 24%
Lamb shoulder, roasted 29%
Lard 99%
Leeks 0%
Lemon 0%
Lemon curd 5%
Lemonade 0%
Lentils 1%
Lettuce 1%
Liver, lamb's, fried 14%
Liver, pig's, braised 8%
Lobster 3%
Low fat spread 40%
Luncheon meat 27%
Lychees 0%
Macadamia nuts 73%
Mackerel 11%
Mackerel flesh, raw 16%
Mackerel, fillet, smoked 13%
Malt loaf 3%
Malted milk drink 7%
Mandarin oranges 0%
Mango 0%
Margarine, low fat 40%
Margarine, very low fat 25%
Margarine, full fat, hard and soft 81%
Margarine, full fat, polyunsaturated 81%
Marmalade 0%

Marrow 0%
Marzipan 25%
Mayonnaise 79%
Meat pie 24%
Melon, cantaloupe 0%
Melon, honey dew 0%
Milk, condensed 9%
Milk, evaporated 9%
Milk, fresh semi-skimmed 2%
Milk, fresh skimmed 1%
Milk, fresh whole 4%
Milk, skimmed, powder 1%
Mince pie 21%
Mincemeat 4%
Mints 1%
Mixed vegetables (frozen) 0%
Molasses 0%
Mousse (fruit) 7%
Muesli 8%
Mushrooms, fried 22%
Mushrooms, raw 1%
Mussels 2%
Mustard and cress 0%
Mustard 8%
Nectarine 0%
Noodles, egg 2%
Oil, coconut 97%
Oil, corn 97%
Oil, olive 96%
Oil, peanut 96%
Oil, soybean 97%
Oil, sunflower 97%
Okra 0%
Olives (in brine) 11%
Onion, fried 33%
Onion, raw 0%
Orange 0%

Orange juice, unsweetened 0%
Orange squash 0%
Oysters 1%
Pancake 7%
Parsley 0%
Parsnips 0%
Passion fruit 0%
Pasta, boiled 1%
Peach, fresh 0%
Peaches, tinned 0%
Peanut butter 51%
Peanuts, salted 49%
Pear 0%
Peas, frozen 0%
Peas, tinned 0%
Pecans 74%
Pepper, green 0%
Pepper, red 0%
Pickle 0%
Pilchards 5%
Pineapple juice 0%
Pineapple, fresh 0%
Pineapple, tinned 0%
Pitta bread 1%
Plaice, steamed 2%
Plum 0%
Popcorn (no salt or fat added) 5%
Pork chop 18%
Pork leg, roasted 32%
Pork pie 29%
Pork, spareribs 39%
Porridge with water 1%
Port 0%
Potatoes, boiled 0%
Potatoes, deep fried chips 40%
Potatoes, jacket 0%
Potatoes, oven chips 8%

Potatoes, roasted 5%
Potatoes, sweet, baked 0%
Prawns 2%
Prunes 1%
Quiche 28%
Rabbit 8%
Radishes 0%
Raisins 0%
Raspberries 0%
Ratatouille 6%
Red wine 0%
Rhubarb (stewed) 0%
Rice, brown, boiled 1%
Rice, white, boiled 0%
Runner beans 0%
Salad dressing: French 39%
Salad dressing: French, low cal 4%
Salad dressing: Italian 60%
Salad dressing: Italian, low cal 5%
Salad dressing: mayonnaise, low calorie 12%
Salad dressing: mayonnaise: 75%
Salami 47%
Salmon, fresh 13%
Salmon, tinned 8%
Sardines 14%
Sausages, beef, grilled 21%
Sausages, pork, grilled 30%
Scampi 21%
Scotch egg 21%
Sesame seeds, dry, hulled 55%
Sherry 0%
Shortbread 26%
Smoked haddock 1%
Smoked salmon 4%
Soy sauce 1%
Soybean curd (tofu) 6%
Spinach 1%

Sponge pudding 16%
Spring greens 0%
Squid 1%
Steak, grilled 6%
Steak and kidney pie 21%
Steak pudding 12%
Stock cube 3%
Strawberries 0%
Stuffing, sage and onion 0%
Sugar, demerara 0%
Sugar, muscavado 0%
Sugar, white 0%
Sultanas 0%
Sunflower seed kernels, dry, hulled 48%
Swede 0%
Sweet potato 1%
Sweetcorn 1%
Sweets, boiled 0%
Swiss roll 5%
Syrup, cane and maple 0%
Taco shell, fried tortilla 19%
Tangerine 0%
Taramasalata 46%
Tartar sauce 59%
Tea 0%
Tinned fruit salad 0%
Toffee apple 0%
Toffees 17%
Tomato, fried 6%
Tomato juice 0%
Tomato paste 0%
Tomato puree 0%
Tomato, raw 0%
Tomato soup 3%
Tomatoes, tinned 0%
Tonic water 0%
Treacle 0%

Tripe, stewed 4%
Trout 5%
Tuna fish tinned in oil 22%
Turkey, roast 10%
Turnip 0%
Veal 28%
Vegetable soup 1%
Venison 6%
Vinegar 0%
Walnuts 52%
Water biscuits 13%
Water chestnuts 1%
Watercress 0%
Watermelon 0%
White wine 0%
Whitebait 48%
Wine, dessert (port, madeira, sweet sherry) 0%
Wine, table (burgundy, rose, white, dry sherry) 0%
Yam 0%
Yeast extract (Marmite) 0%
Yoghurt, fruit (low-fat) 1%
Yoghurt, plain (low-fat) 1%
Yoghurt, soya 2%

## 3. Prepare Food Carefully To Reduce The Risk Of Infection And To Preserve The Vitamin Content

Your body's immune system needs supplies of vitamins and minerals in order to function effectively. In particular, in order to help build up your immune system and fight off infections and cancer your body needs regular supplies of foods which contain antioxidants (beta-carotene, vitamin C and vitamin E) and other substances.

The modern 'meat, butter, cheese, milk' diet is death to your body's immune system not just because those foods are rich in fat but also because they don't contain much in the way of immune-boosting vitamins and minerals.

The healthiest, safest, most efficient and most effective way to obtain the vitamins and minerals you need is to get them from the food you eat. If you eat a good diet you won't have to worry about recommended daily allowances (RDAs) or which sort of supplements to buy.

Your body will get the vitamins and minerals it needs to keep your immune system healthy if you eat a diet which is rich in vegetables, fruits and grains.

However, it is vital to be aware that vitamins can easily be destroyed. Mushrooms, lettuce, broccoli, asparagus and strawberries, for example, all lose their vitamins very quickly. Food which has to be cooked should be cooked for the shortest possible time and at the lowest possible temperature.

In order to ensure that the food you eat retains a high vitamin content – and to minimise the risk of acquiring an infection from your food – you should follow these simple rules:

♦ Food processing tends to reduce the nutritional quality of food and so where possible you should try to buy fresh food and either eat it raw (if appropriate) or eat it after cooking for the shortest length of time.

♦ Buy vegetables whole. Don't have the leaves removed from carrots or the stalk removed from a cabbage or cauliflower. If you buy the vegetable whole vitamin C will continue to be produced and moved into the edible parts of the plant.

♦ Cook foods in the minimum amount of water or steam.

♦ Avoid high cooking temperatures and long heat exposure.

♦ Do not allow food to stand for long periods at room temperature. Do not store food in warm places.

♦ Do not soak vegetables for long periods.

♦ Do not peel fruit or vegetables unless necessary. (For example, do not peel apples or skin potatoes).

♦ Try to use food the day you have bought it rather than use frozen foods. Use foods the day you buy them to get the best out of them.

♦ You can keep fresh products for longer by freezing as soon as you buy them. Deep freezing preserves vitamins and other nutrients. Vegetables should be blanched before freezing. Put them in hot water for a short time. This inactivates enzymes which might otherwise degrade vitamin C.

♦ Make sure that your fridge is kept cold enough. The temperature inside your fridge should be below 3 degrees Centigrade.

♦ Make sure that you wash your hands thoroughly before preparing food. Staphylococcus, for example, can be transmitted hand to hand.

♦ Never re-freeze food which has been previously frozen and then thawed. Thawing increases the number of bacteria and re-freezing food increases the chances of infection.

♦ If you eat meat make sure that it is completely thawed before you start to cook it. If you do not do this then the chances are that the middle of the meat will still be frozen when you start to cook it – and will not be properly cooked when the rest of the meat is ready. Meat which is raw will probably be full of bugs.

♦ Keep foods apart from one another in your fridge in order to reduce the risk of cross contamination. Put meat (a high risk source of infection) at the bottom of the fridge and keep it away from other foods.

♦ Don't ever buy tins which are rusty, bulging or badly damaged.

♦ Always check the sell by date before buying food. Don't be tempted to buy (or use) food which has passed its sell by date.


## 4. Buy Organic Food Whenever Possible

I recommend that whenever possible you purchase 'organic' produce which has been prepared without chemicals.

Nearly half of all the food sold in supermarkets and stores – including fruits, vegetables, bread and meat – contains potentially dangerous pesticide residues. Some chemicals are sprayed onto foods which have grown and which are being picked or shipped to the stores but many chemicals are absorbed when foods are growing and obviously cannot be removed by washing or scraping. Some of the chemicals used by modern farmers are known to cause cancer, asthma and a wide variety of other serious disorders.

Meat is contaminated partly because of the chemicals which are given to animals (to keep them 'healthy' and to make them grow more speedily) and partly because of the chemicals which are put into or onto the food they eat.

Organic food is grown without the use of artificial fertilizers and pesticides and the extra money you have to pay for such food is extremely well spent. Organic farmers use natural fertilisers (such as animal manure and seaweed) and rely on natural biological pest controllers, though some use natural plant based pesticides.

Moreover organic farmers also grow crops in rotation so that their soil is kept in good condition. Growing the same crop year after year in the same massive field probably makes good commercial sense but it means that the food produced will probably be lower in nutritional value.

Organic food is often more expensive than food grown with the aid of large quantities of chemicals simply because farmers who use artificial fertilisers and chemicals to kill bugs, insects and infections can produce bigger, more reliable, more uniform, more predictable and more attractive looking crops. Organic farmers, who have to rely on growing food the way nature intended, tend to have smaller crops and they are more likely to lose their crop through disease.

When buying food and looking for organic produce you should check labels carefully and make sure that you find good, reliable local suppliers. Many organic farmers sell their produce direct to the public and there are now many shops selling organic produce, either as an alternative to food grown with the aid of chemicals or alongside such produce.

In my opinion it is also well worthwhile looking for flour which has been ground in a traditional stone grinding mill. Modern steel rollers, used to crush wheat germ, creates a great deal of destructive heat; natural oils are removed and essential vitamins and minerals which are lost have to be added artificially. An old fashioned, slowing turning millstone crushes the wheat germ slowly – and without it overheating.

## 5. Don't Drink Unfiltered Tap Water

You should drink six to eight decent sized glasses of water a day. Fizzy drinks and caffeinated teas and coffees don't count. Nor do alcoholic drinks. If you can't bear the idea of drinking that much water look for drinks that contain no alcohol, no caffeine and no sugar or sodium. Herbal, fruit or mint teas are fine as are decaffeinated drinks. Alternatively, you can try drinking pure fruit juice diluted with water.

If you want to drink plain water I suggest you avoid tap water. In most countries governments make sure that tap water is regulated and undergoes rigorous tests which means, I'm afraid, that it is pretty much undrinkable and best used for doing the washing up unless you use a filter. Bottled drinking water isn't necessarily pure. Some 'spring water' has been purified or chemically treated while the stuff sold as 'table water' may be nothing more than filtered tap water.

The best bet is probably 'natural mineral water' which comes from a protected, pure, unadulterated source and should not have been treated or tampered with. Natural mineral water may contain some bacteria (though not usually enough to do you any harm) and so you shouldn't keep bottled natural mineral water lying around once the bottle has been opened.

# 6. Improve The Way You Deal With Stress

The evidence shows that the kinder and more thoughtful you are, the more your immune system is likely to be damaged. Worries of any kind can cause serious damage.

We live in a world which is already complex and which is getting steadily more complex by the day. I believe that the conditions which we often describe as anxiety and 'depression' (along with some other troublesome and significant mental disorders) frequently develop because the individual concerned can no longer cope with the barrage of pressures and problems to which they are repeatedly subjected.

Expectations are raised and then left unfulfilled. Feelings of pointlessness and a sense of general despair about the way the world is going are commonplace.

Frustrations, disappointments, 'toxic stresses' and an apparently unending sequence of problems over which the individual has little or no control are common causes of the condition now often officially (and profitably) labelled as 'depression'.

The first step should be to examine and dissect a 'depression' (or anxiety state) so that instead of struggling vainly to tackle a vague, amorphous, ill defined sense of 'depression' it is possible to assess all the influences and factors which might be responsible for the 'depression' and to then tackle each specific cause of the unhappiness.

Understanding what has gone on may lead to a non pharmacological cure for anxiety and 'depression' which will work far more effectively than drugs (and last longer) because it offers a fundamental solution which strikes at the very root of the problem instead of merely papering over the cracks.

## Learn to pay attention

If you learn to pay attention to each moment in your life then you will get far more from your life. You will be living your life to the full and far better able to take advantage of every opportunity and experience which comes your way.

By experiencing each moment in your life with some intensity you will also become far more aware of the ways in which you are damaging your physical and mental health.

Instead of meandering through life in a job you hate or a relationship which isn't ever going to give you any real satisfaction (and ending up miserable and depressed) you will be far more likely to take action that will liberate yourself and allow yourself to live your life to the full.

Many people go through life hardly ever getting out of first gear. They meander along from day to day, hardly ever truly awake and aware of what is going on around them. Only on rare and special occasions (such as the death of someone significant or a birthday, wedding or funeral) do they wake up and become alert and alive.

Because they go through life without really waking up to what is going on around them such individuals ignore the messages their bodies give them.

They never listen to their bodies and so never take advantage of their body's self healing powers.

Your life will become more intense and more enjoyable if you learn to pay complete attention to each moment. Consciously and knowingly experience where you are, what you do and how you feel. Let yourself go. Don't worry about trying to control the present or the future.

We are often encouraged to think that we will be happy when something happens in the future. We decide that we will be happy when we give up the job we hate, when the kids leave home, when we get a promotion, when we lose weight, when the business begins to take off, when we have a new car and so on.

But if you are constantly postponing happiness when will you ever give yourself a chance to be happy?

Life is only really present in the here and now. Life isn't in the future because the future isn't yet here. And it isn't in the past because the past is gone.

But be warned.

Once you become aware of your life – and the way you are living it – you may need to make changes.

We often shut off our awareness of the world outside because we simply can't bear the reality which surrounds us.

When you become truly aware of the world around you then you may suddenly discover that you have acquired the strength to stand up for yourself, to turn away from bad relationships or to leave a job you hate.

## There's More To Life Than Having Everything

We have more 'things' and more 'comfort' than any other civilisation in history. But 'depression' and unhappiness are probably commoner than in any other civilisation.

Our society values material acquisitions more than anything else. We are taught that we will only find contentment by increasing our level of consumption.

Happiness comes with a bigger house, a bigger car and more expensive clothes.

And so we are pushed to go through our lives acquiring expensive 'stuff' which we may neither really need nor truly want. Our goals become materialistic instead of personal.

We forget to live because we believe that we will only truly be happy when we have achieved another goal. But when will we know when we have enough? Will $50,000 be enough? What about $500,000? $5,000,000? $ 50,000,000?

And if we are driven only by the happiness we think we will find when we have reached a certain goal what will we have to look forward if we ever do have enough? (And if we admit that we will never have enough then we are admitting that we are dooming ourselves to permanent disappointment and frustration.)

As a wise man once said: 'There must be more to life than having everything.'

## Protect Yourself From Misery

I have given up watching the TV news. And I only rarely buy newspapers. I no longer expose myself to a daily diet of misery. This is not because I am disinterested in the problems of the world – I fight for the things I believe in and I read enough news magazines and news agency summaries to know about the important things going on in the world. But I know that I can only cope with so much misery and sadness.

I protect myself because if I allowed myself to be subjected to a constant daily diet of misery and horror I would not be able to cope – or have the strength to fight for the things in which I believe.

I don't know whether there is any more violence or horror in the world today than there was five hundred years ago. I suspect not. But that is an academic and irrelevant question. The point is that modern communications methods make these horrors available to us all on an hourly basis. At any one time there are around forty wars going on around the world. All these wars – and the accompanying horrors – are brought into our homes through the magic of television.

Modern communications techniques mean that you and I receive more information every day than our ancestors had to cope with in years.

The modern media enables us to expose ourselves to many horrors and injustices about which we can do nothing. Television gives us instant access to other people's pain.

But however much we care we can't fight against every injustice in the world.

I believe that one of the reasons why so many people do not seem to care these days is that they are protecting themselves by deliberately staying aloof and not allowing themselves to respond to what they hear about.

People numb themselves and suppress their emotions in order to survive.

They become unfeeling because they are overexposed to horror and they simply cannot cope. They close their eyes and their hearts to protect themselves (and because the horrors they see and hear about are endless they do not believe they can do anything that will make a difference).

If you want to stay alert but sensitive to the world's problems then I suggest that you too limit your exposure to news programmes.

Limiting your exposure to the daily diet of horror and injustice will enable you to retain the strength to do what you can to fight for truth and justice.

## What Do You Really Want?

Do you know what makes you happy? Do you know when you are happy? How many moments of happiness did you have last week?

You have to make time for happiness. You have to be ready for it. And you have to work at it.

When the good times come you have to make a real effort to enjoy them; to look around and take notice of the world so that you can savour and remember your happiness (and use it to keep you going when the times get rough).

Ask yourself these four simple questions – you might find the answers illuminating.

What in your life gives you most fun? How much time do you spend doing it?

What in your life gives you least enjoyment? How much time do you spend doing that?

Another question to ask yourself is 'Why?'

Why do you want a better job? Why do you want to save money? Why do you want to move house? Why do you want to buy a holiday home?

Only when you ask yourself 'Why?' will you know what you really need and what you are prepared to do for it.

Most people earn and spend without ever asking themselves 'Why?' They blindly sell their time (which is the same as selling their lives) for money which they spend on things they neither want nor need.

Ask yourself 'Why?' more often and you will learn more about yourself and what you are doing.

But be warned. Asking yourself this simple question can be unnerving.

You may get answers.

And if you have been going through life for years without knowing where you were headed (or why) then you may find the answers you get rather startling.

Assess all the influences on your life and ask yourself how these things contribute to your life and potential for enjoyment and satisfaction.

Consider each influence and ask yourself: 'Should I discard it or give it more of my energy?'

## Protest And Preserve Yourself

Finally, here are some simple, specific ways to help protect and preserve your immune system.

♦ Be prepared to admit when you're feeling tired. If you keep going when you're exhausted you'll not only make yourself worse (by doing further damage to your immune system) but you'll also let yourself – and the people around you – down. You can't do your best work when you're suffering from burn out.

♦ Learn to manage your time as efficiently as possible. Plan your day. Keep a diary so that important engagements and commitments don't suddenly creep up on you.

♦ If you feel ill take time off. Don't think that you're indispensable and must carry on. The cemeteries are full of people who thought they were indispensable but life goes on without them. If you feel exhausted then your body is telling you that it needs to rest. Remember that regular holidays are important – and make sure that the holiday you choose is relaxing! Your immune system will automatically repair and rebuild itself when you take a break.

♦ If your life is full of battles and arguments make sure that you take time out to relax and enjoy yourself. And make sure that you differentiate between those battles which are worth fighting and those which are merely adding to the stress in your life. If you learn to walk away from trivial and insignificant problems you will retain your strength for the battles which really matter. Stand up for yourself over important issues but be prepared to walk away from arguments when the underlying issue isn't truly important. People who are always complaining burn themselves out with anger so think very carefully before allowing yourself to get heated up. If the battle is important then do what you think is right – and fight to the last breath if necessary. If the battle isn't important then try to shrug your shoulders and walk away.

♦ Make sure that you get enough sleep. If you have difficulty in relaxing at night try having a hot bath before you go to bed. Don't do any work for at least an hour before you try to get to sleep. Watch a relaxing video or read an amusing or entertaining book. Poor sleep is a symptom of burn out – and it makes things steadily worse. Your immune system gets recharged while you're sleeping – as long as you are relaxed.

♦ Learn to say 'no' more often. Don't let yourself be tricked into taking on too many responsibilities by people who know how to make you feel guilty! Get your priorities sorted out and remember that you – and your family and friends – need some of your life.

♦ Try not to get too upset when things go wrong. Remember that you can't get anywhere in life without taking risks or without making mistakes. Try not to brood over your failures but try to learn from your mistakes. Otherwise your bad days will smoulder and add to your burn out.

♦ Do you touch the people you love often enough? If your immune system is being damaged by stress – then the chances are high that you touch the people you love far too little. And you probably need to give out more cuddles too.

Touching – and being touched – will help improve the effectiveness of your immune system and increase your body's resistance to infection and cancer.

Ask yourself how many times you've hugged the people who are closest to you in the last 24 hours. And ask yourself how often you've touched the people you love.

If you don't touch or hug or cuddle people often it may be that you have to battle against a long established feeling that such outward signs of affection are wrong.

If your parents didn't hug or cuddle you very often you may find it difficult to let yourself go.

You may have even been encouraged to believe that hugging, cuddling and touching are embarrassing or too 'showy'.

Boys are often told off for wanting a hug.

'You're too old for that sort of thing,' Father will say because he feels uncomfortable at the prospect of close physical contact.

If you think that you need to touch – and be touched – more often make today the day you start:

♦ When you greet a loved one – even if its only after a few hours parting – put an arm around them. You don't have to start with a full blooded hug if that makes you feel embarrassed. Build up to a hug slowly!

♦ When you're leaving someone – again if its only for a few hours – touch them on the arm or shoulder. Try a peck on the cheek if you're shy about a full mouth to mouth kiss. Again, build up to a proper cuddle.

♦ When you kiss someone 'hello' or 'goodbye' don't be content with a distant peck on the cheek. Put your arms around them, give them a big hug.

♦ When you greet close friends get into the habit of touching them – maybe clasping their hands or forearm, or perhaps putting an arm around them.

Hugging, touching and kissing aren't just for lovers. If you regularly hug, touch and kiss all the people who matter to you then you'll feel better – and so will they!

## 7. General Advice

### Don't Be Too Obsessed With Cleanliness

Have you ever wondered whether the modern obsession with hygiene could have possibly made us more susceptible to illness? Poor living conditions are known to be a significant factor in the development of many diseases (for example tuberculosis) but could too much of a good thing be a bad thing? There is growing evidence to show that it could.

Research has now shown that the level of pollutants (such as dangerous gases) is usually higher in the home than outside it. This is true even in the most polluted cities. Two environmental engineers working at the University of Texas in Austin, US have recently suggested that by trying to keep our homes clean we may be creating more pollution. Baths, showers, washing machines and dishwashers can all be serious sources of pollution because they extract small amounts of chemicals from the water they use and push those chemicals out into the air. Most public water supplies contain small amounts of toxic chemicals (mostly these are the remains of chemicals used in the chlorination process) and these chemicals are released when the water is heated and splashed about a good deal. It appears that a dishwasher is particularly good at extracting toxic chemicals from tap water but even a shower head can do quite a job of this.

Children who live in an unhealthily artificial (and clean) environment, and who have very little contact with infective organisms, may grow up without having acquired the immunity which might help protect them from some infections later in life.

And children who 'miss' common childhood illnesses (such as the big four: measles, rubella, mumps and chickenpox) may suffer far more seriously if they get those infections when they are adults.

Too much cleanliness may result in an increased susceptibility to infection and in addition some immunologists now believe that the dramatic increase in allergy problems such as asthma, eczema and hayfever in recent years may be due to excessive hygiene.

Modern babies have very little contact with mycobacteria (which live in soil and streams) and this could result in their immune systems becoming too quick to develop allergy responses (as well as too slow to kill bacteria and viruses).

It's too early to offer definitive advice on this just yet. But my instinct tells me that children just might grow up stronger, healthier and less likely to develop allergies if they spent more time playing in the garden and less time living in a sterile antiseptic-soaked environment.

If I'm right doctors and drug companies will probably soon find a way of cashing in on this. What odds against the next generation of doctors prescribing 'mud pie dabbling' three times a week? The mud pies will, of course, come courtesy of the pharmaceutical industry. They will be expensively pre-packed and guaranteed to contain just the right number of mycobacteria.

Meanwhile, a tad more soil, a dab more mud and a spray or two less of antiseptic may be a wise move.

## Minimise Your Risk Of Being Made Ill By Electricity

♦ Don't have mains powered radios, answering machines, clocks or other electrical devices unnecessarily close to you – on your desk, in the kitchen or by your bed. Battery operated appliances are probably safer.

♦ Don't sit within two and a half or three feet of the front, sides or the back of a Visual Display Unit on a computer or word processor.

♦ If you are pregnant try to keep away from Visual Display Units completely. A study of over 1,500 women showed that pregnant women who spend more than 20 hours a week working on such terminals have a greater chance of having a miscarriage.

♦ If your child's school is within 150 yards of a major electricity supply line ask the authorities to test the electrical fields in classrooms, playground and sports fields.

♦ Don't sit (and don't let children sit) closer than three feet from your television set when it is switched on. TV sets produce potentially dangerous electrical fields which are stronger the closer you get.

♦ Unplug electrical blankets before you get into bed.

♦ Don't sit or stand in front of household appliances such as microwave ovens when they are switched on.

♦ Try not to live in a home within 150 yards of a major electricity supply line. I think this is probably particularly important if you have small children or are pregnant.

## Use Your Mobile Telephone As Safely As Possible

♦ Use your mobile phone only when absolutely necessary – and keep calls as brief as possible. Mobile phones should be used for emergency calls rather than routine calls.

♦ Use the forwarding facility when using the phone indoors. Most mobile phones can be adapted so that callers are re-directed to a landline telephone.

♦ A hands-free kit (with microphone and ear piece) enables mobile phone users to use their telephones without holding them to the side of their heads.

♦ Mobile telephone users can protect themselves by opening a window when using their telephone. I confess that at first reading this sounded to me the sort of thing that might have been put about by James Thurber's aunt (the one who, the American humorist said, claimed that if you didn't put plugs in electrical sockets at night then electricity would dribble out onto the floor). But my scepticism was unfounded. Whenever a mobile phone is switched on it searches for a signal. If the phone can't find a signal it increases its power. Naturally, this means that anything that gets in the way of the signal (such as a plate glass window) will mean that the phone has to use more power. Every mobile phone I've seen comes equipped with a meter which measures and reports the level of the signal. The better the signal the less power the phone will be using – and so the safer it will be. When the signal is poor the health threat is increased. It is clear therefore that anything you can do to reduce the amount of power your phone needs to use in order to work properly will be a help in reducing the health risk. Fitting an external aerial in your car may help. And opening a window (whether you are at home or in a car) may help.

♦ Because of the concern about the risks which may be associated with the use of mobile telephones it is now possible to purchase devices which are designed to help protect the brain from the microwaves being produced. However, some of these devices make a portable telephone heavier, bulkier and more difficult to carry around. There is also a risk that they may have an adverse effect on the telephone's performance. I haven't yet seen any evidence showing that these devices work. But I haven't seen any evidence suggesting that they could be dangerous either. They may be worth using.

♦ One leading car manufacturer now warns customers not to use mobile phones inside cars because of the danger that the electromagnetic fields produced by the phone working within the car's metal shell may be a health hazard.

♦ Possibly the most useful health protection tip I've heard came from the boss of a telephone company. He says he wraps his fingers around his telephone so that the phone itself is always an inch or so away from the side of his head. Not surprisingly this can make it difficult to conduct a conversation if there is a lot of background noise (in a railway station for example) but it does reduce the dose of microwave radiation next to the head.

♦ If for some reason you can't use a hand free microphone and earpiece turn up the volume so that you can hold the phone some distance from your head.

## Watch Out For The Early Warning Signs Of Cancer

♦ Many cancers are curable – especially if caught early. Here are some cancer signs you should watch out for. Remember:
**a)** a patient with cancer may suffer from one, all or none of these symptoms
**b)** this list is not comprehensive (there are other symptoms and signs of cancer)
**c)** a symptom on this list may be caused by something other than cancer. If you are at all worried you should always see your doctor as soon as possible for advice.

♦ Cancer of the large bowel: change in bowel habits (diarrhoea or constipation), unexplained weight loss, pain, passing blood.

♦ Cancer of the cervix: unexplained bleeding or discharge, pain or bleeding after sex, weight loss.

- Cancer of the breast: swelling or lump in breast, bloody discharge from nipple, enlarged glands in armpit, dimpling of the skin of the breast.

- Cancer of the lung: persistent bad cough, blood in sputum, chest pain, wheezing, weight loss.

- Cancer of the stomach: weight loss, persistent indigestion, vomiting blood, lump in abdomen, feeling full after very small meals.

- Cancer of the liver: pain in abdomen, loss of appetite, weight loss, yellow eyes and skin, abdomen swollen.

- Cancer of the ovary: irregular periods, hard lump in abdomen, pain during sex, bowel problems, excessive hair growth, voice gets deeper.

- Cancer of the brain: headaches, vomiting, visual disturbances, weakness or paralysis, dizziness, fits, memory loss, personality changes.

- Cancer of the skin: skin lesion that doesn't heal, bleeds, gets larger, changes shape, size or colour.

- Cancer of the prostate: pain, urine retention, difficulty in passing urine.

- Cancer of the testicle: swelling in testicle.

- Cancer of the blood (leukaemia): tiredness, paleness, bruising, bleeding easily, lots of infections.

- Cancer of the womb: bleeding after sex, lump felt in abdomen.

- Cancer of the throat: hoarseness, lump in throat, difficulty in swallowing, swollen glands in neck.

**Beware of Vaccines**

Many readers who have tried to discuss vaccines with their doctors have complained that their physicians simply insist that vaccines are perfectly safe and that that is the end of the matter.

In my view, everyone should be told the facts so that they

can make up their own minds about the value of any vaccine. Deciding whether or not to have a vaccination is a big decision. It isn't something to be done lightly. The wrong decision can easily lead to a lifetime of regrets. Sadly, however, one big problem is undoubtedly the fact that many doctors simply don't know very much about the safety or effectiveness of vaccines. They know what the government tells them and they know what the company which makes the vaccine tells them. But I don't trust governments and I don't think that companies making vaccines are the right source of unbiased information about effectiveness and safety.

'My doctor implied that I was being stupid when I said I wasn't sure that I wanted my child vaccinated,' complained one reader of mine. 'His attitude was that it had nothing to do with me and that I should allow him to do whatever he thought best.'

'My wife came home crying,' complained another reader. 'She had had the temerity to question her doctor about vaccination. He told her that if she refused to have our child vaccinated he would call in the social workers since in his view our refusal to allow vaccination made us unfit to be parents. What really upset me is that my wife hadn't refused to have our child vaccinated. She just wanted to talk about it.'

This paternalistic attitude seems strong among doctors and other health workers, most of whom seem to prefer to answer any questions with abuse rather than facts.

Before you allow your doctor to vaccinate your child (or you) ask your doctor these essential questions:

♦ How dangerous is the disease for which the vaccine is being given? (Exactly what are the chances that it will kill or cripple?)

♦ How effective is the vaccine?

♦ How dangerous is the vaccine? (Exactly what are the chances that it will kill or cripple?) What side effects are associated with the vaccine?

♦ Which patients should not be given the vaccine?

I advise patients to ask doctors to give them written confirmation that they have personally investigated the risk-benefit ratio of the vaccine and that, having looked at all the evidence, they believe that the vaccine is safe and essential for that particular patient. How could any doctor object to signing such a confirmation?

I cannot give you specific advice about whether or not you should have your child vaccinated against whooping cough, measles or any other disease. It would be dangerous and irresponsible for me to try to offer you specific advice because we are all different and circumstances change from day to day.

My own personal view is that vaccines are unsafe and worthless. I would not allow myself to be vaccinated again and I will in future advise family and friends not to be vaccinated. Readers must, however, make their own judgements based on all the available evidence. I strongly recommend that anyone contemplating vaccination discuss the issue with their own medical adviser.

Infectious diseases are least likely to affect (and to kill) those who have healthy immune systems. I no longer believe that vaccines have any role to play in the protection of the community or the individual. Vaccines may be profitable but, in my view, they are neither safe nor effective. I prefer to put my trust in building up my immune system.

Since vaccines are usually given by injection they by pass the body's normal defence systems (the skin, tonsils and so on). Vaccination is an extremely unnatural process.

I have for many years been concerned about the safety and efficacy of specific vaccines. Those fears have gradually gelled into a general conviction that vaccination programmes are neither sufficiently safe nor sufficiently effective to be acceptable. It is worth remembering that those involved in trying to 'sell' vaccination programmes to the public have repeatedly lied and tried to prevent the publication of the truth.

## Avoid aeroplanes whenever possible

The time has come when we should all question our travel plans a little more closely.

Is your next trip really necessary? And if the trip is necessary would it be possible to make the same journey by train or boat? Some modern trains are 'closed systems' but since doors are opened occasionally there is a decent chance that you might get a little fresh air to breathe occasionally.

## Try to avoid buildings which have closed circuit air conditioning or heating systems

When air is constantly re-circulated your chances of acquiring an infection are dramatically increased. If one person sneezes or coughs then the chances are high that everyone in the building will be exposed to the bug.

## Try to keep away from hospitals, doctors' clinics and other places where sick people congregate

I used to favour open plan wards (as designed by Florence Nightingale) since patients in such wards can be kept constantly under supervision by nurses. The explosion in the incidence of antibiotic-resistant bugs means that single rooms are now preferable for any patient requiring hospital treatment.

## Remember Coleman's first law!

Most doctors prescribe far too many different drugs and as a result they have no idea what side effects are associated with the drugs they are handing out.

You should always remember Coleman's First Law of Modern Medicine: 'If you develop new symptoms while being treated for any medical condition the chances are that the new symptoms are caused by the treatment you are receiving.'

One in six patients in hospital are there because they have been made ill by doctors. The reason is simple. Few doctors know Coleman's First Law of Modern Medicine. You should never forget it. It will be a vital weapon in your armoury in the years ahead.

Never forget that many of the chronically disabling illnesses of the twentieth century are actually caused by drug therapy.

Be wary, too, of taking drugs which aren't essential. For example, if your doctor wants to prescribe an antibiotic ask him if he thinks it is really essential – or if he just giving you the prescription because he thinks you want an antibiotic. Don't take drugs unless you really need them. Ask if there is a non-drug alternative and ask exactly why the drug is being prescribed and what the consequences could be if you don't take it.

In short: don't take drugs (either prescribed or bought over the pharmacy counter) unless you really need them. Always investigate other ways to deal with health problems.